TWINS AND MULTIPLE BIRTHS

TWINS AND MULTIPLE BIRTHS

The Essential Parenting Guide from Pregnancy to Adulthood

Dr Carol Cooper

assisted by TAMBA
(The Twins and Multiple Birth Association)

VERMILION
London

To my family, who are often a challenge
but always an inspiration

1 3 5 7 9 10 8 6 4 2

Text copyright © Dr Carol Cooper 1997
Illustration copyright © Random House UK Ltd 1997

First published in the United Kingdom in 1997 by Vermilion
an imprint of Ebury Press
Random House
20 Vauxhall Bridge Road
London SW1V 2SA

Random House Australia (Pty) Limited
20 Alfred Street, Milsons Point, Sydney,
New South Wales 2061, Australia

Random House New Zealand Limited
18 Poland Road, Glenfield,
Auckland 10, New Zealand

Random House South Africa (Pty) Limited
Endulini, 5A Jubilee Road,
Parktown 2193, South Africa

Random House UK Limited Reg. No. 954009

A CIP catalogue record for this book is available from the British Library

ISBN: 0 09 181471 5

Printed and bound in Great Britain by
Mackays of Chatham, Ltd.

This work cannot be exhaustive, and nothing in it is
intended to be a substitute for consultation with a
medical practitioner or other professionals

CONTENTS

ACKNOWLEDGEMENTS

I am greatly indebted to TAMBA who first agreed that there was a need for this book, and then entrusted me with the task of writing it. It would have perished shortly after the first page without the superb help of their honorary consultants who have provided information and advice, and allowed me access to their work and ideas.

I should particularly like to mention Dr John Buckler, Jane Ellison, Peter Hendy-Ibbs, Rachel Hudson, Judi Linney, Pat Preedy, Audrey Sandbank, Gina Siddons, Jane Spillman and Jill Walton. I am also very grateful to Dr Elizabeth Bryan and MBF for much expertise and support, Professor David Hay and AMBA (Australian Multiple Births Association) who have helped me and allowed me to quote from the La Trobe Study, Professor Jim Stevenson and Dr Peter Tymms. Naturally the comments and interpretation in this book are mine, and are not necessarily endorsed by TAMBA or any other organisation.

Many twins, triplets and their families have been kind enough to let me repeat their spontaneous words and innermost thoughts. In all, a great many people have helped to stimulate me and shape my thinking, and to turn what started as parenting into a lifelong interest as well as an adventure. I hope I have not left anyone out.

Carol Cooper

FOREWORD

The publication of this new book on the subject of twins and higher multiple births is very welcome, as parents and professionals always need up-to-date information. When TAMBA (or as it was known then – TCA – Twins Club Association) was formed in 1978, very few books existed on the care and upbringing of children who were born as twins, triplets, or more. Those that had been published were sadly outdated and generally from overseas. They included practices which were not understood by parents in the UK and terms which were certainly unfamiliar to many.

In the years since TAMBA's formation that situation has changed and many excellent books have been written and published from the UK perspective. However, it has been several years since a new, practical book has come on to the market. The 'world' of multiple births has changed, like so many other areas. TAMBA is aware of the immense practical, financial and emotional needs of multiple-birth families. The medical world has influenced the development of new and exciting techniques, many of which have directly impacted upon the area of multiple births. Medical and technological advancement has ensured that far more babies born as a result of a multiple conception can survive. In addition, more parents who were previously unable to conceive are now facing a more positive outcome in their endeavours to become parents – although, sadly not all – and many of these are having twins, triplets or more! This has resulted in a greater increase in multiple births, and studies have indicated that few doctors and nurses realise what is involved in looking after and relating to two or more babies.

Dr Carol Cooper has written her book to provide a modern outlook to modern situations. She has provided a frank look at issues which, in earlier years, were not discussed with prospective or expecting parents. Many things known only to the medical profession – and even then only to those directly involved in the specialist care of such pregnancies – are now in the public domain. Like medical advancement, information given to parents is more detailed and more frank.

Dr Cooper has produced a book that is easy to read, more appropriate to the busy parent of twins or more, and one which can be referred to at varying stages of the parents' and children's development. Whilst most of the readers will be mothers, I am sure that many fathers and carers will want to pick up the book to read about what will happen to them next!

The book starts with a punchy introduction, leading the reader to realise that the rest of the contents will be accessible and worthy of frequent breaks in routine to find out more. The chapters follow a natural progression through the life cycle of all multiple-birth families – from preconception through to the later years of child rearing. It has often been said that rearing twins or more never gets easier, just different! This book highlights this basic fact, although one must not forget that having two, three or more babies at once is special and that, whilst incredibly exhausting in the early months, it can lead to many pleasures that those blessed with children born at different times cannot hope to achieve.

This book will be valuable, as it gives a comprehensive overview of the practical management of children born two, three or more together.

Jane Ellison
TAMBA Chairman
1997

INTRODUCTION

Since certain topics have universal appeal, I should mention at the outset that this book is going to be about sex and money. Twins and higher multiples usually start off with sex, and always cost a lot of money.

When I was expecting my twins, I realized how much the processes of childbirth and parenting are geared towards having merely one baby at once. It was intensely frustrating to read about breast-feeding or bonding when no thought had been given to the fact that, for many mothers, their baby was planning to arrive in the world with at least one companion.

I was fortunate to make contact early on with the Twins and Multiple Births Association (TAMBA), which was founded in 1978 and supports families with multiples through local twins' clubs and major specialist support groups. I learned a lot and forged lasting friendships. I also met Dr Elizabeth Bryan, who is widely regarded as the leading paediatrician in the care of multiples. My twins attended her first twins' clinic at Queen Charlotte's Hospital in January 1987, and the whole family has kept in close touch with her and the Multiple Births Foundation (MBF), which she launched in 1988 to provide support for families with multiples and professionals who care for them.

Although very different, both organizations also play a part in promoting public and professional awareness of the needs of multiples. If my own experience is anything to go by, awareness is much needed because most of the population is unenlightened and some even appear incapable of simple arithmetic. One mother of four, who should have known

better, asked me whether having twins was any different
from having one baby. An otherwise intelligent friend commented sceptically, 'If having twins or triplets is as difficult
as you make out, why do people always say how lucky you
are?' Outside the school gates, another mother opined that
having twins was so much easier than having one at a time.
According to her logic, life with quads would have been a
doddle.

When you have twins, everyone around you is ecstatic.
You're thrilled too. Or are you? If you don't already have
children, you may not be over the moon at the prospect of
an instant family and might have preferred to be broken in
gently, like most parents. If you already have one child or
more, you may find yourself even more short of arms and
time. People admire twins and strangers stop to chat, but
rarely offer help, and sometimes, worn out by the demands of
intensive baby care, I went green with envy at the sight of
mothers with singletons.

The reasons are simple. With twins, whatever one baby
needs, the other may need too, and more or less at the same
time! Twin pregnancies are more demanding physically and
often mentally, and twin births of necessity, have a higher
rate of medical intervention. Because they are more likely to
be premature or small, many babies born as multiples are
admitted to the special care unit. Later, their parents face
exhaustion from disruptive sleep patterns, the challenge of
feeding two babies at once, the logistics of getting about, and
the extra energy required in the rearing of more than one child
at a time. Many mothers revel in these challenges, while
others may find solutions elusive.

As I learned more about multiples both from a practical
point of view, as a parent, and from a medical angle, as a GP,
I realized that things could have worked out better for some
parents of twins had they taken a different approach early on.
Many mothers, charmed by the notion of twins, may focus

too much on the children's twin-ness, to the detriment of their development and sometimes of the other siblings' well-being too. With some juggling, parents can manage multiples, but what happens to the rest of the family? It takes skill and insight to balance the needs of twins with those of the other members of the household.

I found several excellent books on multiples, but some of those written from a parent's standpoint were getting a bit out of date and I wanted to remedy that. In so doing I was conscious, as I was in my work as a doctor, that the advice one so willingly dishes out may not be suitable for everyone. This was very clear to me from the writings of some general childcare experts, and I got particularly fed up with the view that going back to work was something a few mothers had to do through lack of choice. This is increasingly untrue since these days many mothers feel morally obliged to work, and others just want to.

There are many other areas where one author's ideal strategy can easily become a tyranny for others to follow. Society is hard enough as it is on imperfect mothers and I feel strongly about the one or two manuals which dictate to parents, making them suspect they are deficient unless they do everything in a certain way, or feel particular emotions for their children.

When a couple have children, they inevitably go through life-style changes. These are particularly marked when they have multiples. I have tried to address these changes. But in writing this book I wanted to share with readers not so much my own philosophy but my experience and medical knowledge. Even if you are a first-time parent, you will have your own approach and will soon learn to trust your own instincts rather than mine. In parenting, the road you travel is a rocky one. Some of the route is well marked but the rest is largely uncharted territory. If you are new to parenting as well as to twins, it's practically a foreign country. This book describes the parenting journey as accurately as I could make it. I have made use of many people's maps and illustrated it with jottings from other travellers. I hope it points out some of the delights of the scenery as well as a few of the pitfalls to be avoided.

One final note: in common with other childcare manuals, this book follows the convention of female parent with male infant. This, of course, is done for the sake of clarity.

Chapter One

IN THE BEGINNING

Multiple births began to decline in the 1970s but, thanks to social changes and medical advances (explored later in this chapter), are now on the way up again. In the last decade there has been a dramatic increase, so that the incidence of twins is one set for every 76 live births. In 1995, 8749 sets of twins were born in England and Wales. Meanwhile, the incidence of triplets has trebled in little more than nine years: 282 new sets of triplets were born in England and Wales in 1995 and, incidentally, seven sets of quads.

Higher multiples are much less common, but they do occur. The highest recorded order is believed to be nonuplets, born to Mrs Geraldine Brodrick in Sydney, Australia, in June 1971. But her nine babies (four girls and five boys) survived only a few days.

Perhaps because twins are fascinating, there have been many misconceptions about them. According to beliefs held at various times, twins have been thought to represent good luck or fertility, to be infertile themselves or, in the case of boy girl pairs, to have indulged in an incestuous relationship in the womb. In medieval Europe especially, a woman bearing twins was thought to have had an adulterous liaison, which indeed she may have done.

Several mythological and religious figures have been twins, such as the Greek gods Castor and Pollux, the biblical pair Jacob and Esau, the Scandinavian gods Hoder and Balder, and Romulus and Remus, abandoned to be brought up by a she-wolf. Famous twins include Carol and Mark Thatcher and June and Jennifer Gibbons (the silent twins of

Marjorie Wallace's book of the same name). Several appear to have made their twinship work for them. The identical twins Ross and Norris McWhirter, for example, were able sportsmen as well as co-writers of *The Guinness Book of Records*, and Peter and Michael Ball were bishops of two dioceses. The best-known lone twin is probably Elvis Presley, but there is also Liberace, who was born Wladziu Valentino in Milwaukee, Wisconsin, in May 1919 weighing nearly 6 kg (13 lbs), while his brother was stillborn.

· *Types of twins* ·

Your own twins may never achieve fame or notoriety, but they will be special and are bound to attract attention. One of the first questions you are likely to be asked is, 'Are they identical?'

Pretty well everyone nowadays knows that there are two kinds of twin – identical and non-identical – though they don't always understand what causes the two types.

Identical twins develop from the splitting of a single zygote or fertilized egg, and are often referred to as monozygotic (MZ) or monovular twins. These twins almost always look very similar and, in true Enid Blyton fashion, can often play successful practical jokes on the unsuspecting. Identical twins are always the same sex, a fact which Shakespeare failed to appreciate when he wrote the indistinguishable Viola and Sebastian into *Twelfth Night*, though since he had a boy–girl pair himself he should perhaps have realized it. Identicals can only be of different sex if something goes slightly awry at the time of cleavage of the egg, so that one of the X chromosomes goes missing. This is extremely unusual.

Non-identical twins are about twice as common as identical (MZ) twins, and are no more alike (or dissimilar) in looks and personality than any other two siblings. They are conceived by the union of two different sperms with two separate eggs, so they arise from two fertilized eggs (zygotes) and are also called dizygotic (DZ), binovular, or fraternal twins.

Since one sperm may carry an X chromosome and the other a Y, DZ twins can be of different sexes and in fact about half of them are. Since two-thirds of all twins are DZ and one half of these are boy–girl pairs, in total a third of all twins are mixed-sex pairs.

DZ twins share half of their genes, on average. Sometimes it's more, sometimes less, which explains why some non-identicals are very similar while others are not at all. They need not have the same father. In 1978, a young German woman gave birth to non-identical boys, one of whom was white and the other black, both conceived on the same day by different men. It is not very unusual to find twins of apparently different race. The likeliest cause is not promiscuity, but simply that one or other parent is of mixed racial origin and thus offers a rich pool of genes for their children to draw on.

DZ twins are not necessarily conceived on the same day. They can be conceived several days apart, in a phenomenon called superfecundation. This occurs because a woman can be fertile for several days in each menstrual cycle. Perhaps this is why couples with more active sex lives are likelier to have twins.

DZ twins can also be implanted into the womb at different times, sometimes two or more years apart in the case of assisted-fertility techniques whereby one embryo is frozen for later use. These are twins only in the sense that they were conceived together; they are no more alike than if they had been conceived at different times. At Bourn Hall Fertility Clinic, Cambridge, two embryos from the same woman were implanted two years apart into different surrogate mothers, making medical history and resulting in what the tabloid papers have called 'time-warp twins'. However, few parents would probably think of them as twins because caring for them is little different from bringing up two singletons.

The third type of twin is sometimes called dispermatic. In most Western countries, about a third of all twins are identical while two-thirds are non-identical, but there is almost certainly a third type, created when one egg splits into two and then each half, so to speak, is fertilized by separate sperms. In this case the mother's contribution to the genes of the twins is the same, but the father's may be different for each twin. Since the father's chromosomes determine an offspring's gender, these twins could in theory be of different sexes.

This type of twin is known to occur in other mammals. If the phenomenon occurs in humans, one might expect the twins to be a little more alike than many fraternal twins, but less alike than identical twins. It's not at all clear how common this third type might be, but some twins, mine included, like to believe they were conceived this way. What they most enjoy is the puzzled look people give them when they claim to be 'half-identical'.

· *What Causes Twins?* ·

There has been a great deal of research into this question, especially over the last twenty years, but the full answer is still not known. In the case of DZ twins, science has highlighted a few factors, including:

- race
- family history
- the mother's age
- how many children she has already had
- her height
- increased fertility
- decreased fertility (if treated).

While the incidence of MZ twins is fairly constant at about 3.5 per 1000 maternities (or completed pregnancies), there is a wide geographical variation in the rate of DZ twinning.

Some parts of Africa enjoy the highest rate of twinning. Compared with her English counterpart, a Nigerian woman is about four times more likely to have twins, whereas in South-East Asia in general, and Japan in particular, DZ twinning rates are low, although this is changing because of social changes including fertility treatment. The rate for MZ twins is on a par with those of the UK.

Locality is important within the UK too, though to a lesser degree. Analysis by TAMBA has shown that in the North of England, women have fewer multiples. In Tyne and Wear, for instance, the average rate in 1992 was 9.83 multiple births per 1000 maternities. Surrey, on the other hand, saw an average of 14.89 per 1000 maternities. This may be related to the availability of treatment for fertility problems, as well as the fact that in the South-East mothers tend to be older than those in the North. There are small scattered areas where twins seem especially common, but this is usually no more than one might expect by chance; there is no real evidence for 'something in the water', as locals claim.

Non-identical twins often run in families. They are sometimes said to skip a generation, from grandmother to granddaughter, but this isn't true. All it means is that a family history of twins can make them a lot more likely — but not inevitable. If you are a twin yourself, have twin siblings, or have already had one set of twins, your chances of having non-identical (DZ) twins are several times higher than the average woman's. Some couples with this sort of pedigree like to insure against the possibility of twins. Eagle Star is one company that offers multiple-birth insurance, paying out several thousand pounds if the woman has twins, but the policy has to be taken out before the eleventh week of pregnancy and there are restrictions as to who is eligible for cover.

It's the mother's side of the family that matters in determining how many eggs a woman produces. After all, men don't ovulate. And in each ejaculate a man produces between 150 million and a billion sperms, far more than are needed to sire just two babies.

These statements demonstrate some of the ignorance that still surrounds twinning. In fact, the father does seem to make a contribution, so men's bar-room boasts about producing twins may be rooted in reality after all. There is a classic Russian tale about Vassilief, a man who had two wives in succession and fathered a total of 84 children, amongst them four sets of quads and seven sets of triplets. Now, science tells us, sperm may do something to the ovum which makes it more likely to split. Perhaps this explains the occasional family in which identical twins seem to be passed on via the male line.

Both the main types of twin may run in families, though it's not certain how. New research from Sweden shows that any mother who is a twin herself – either MZ or DZ – runs a higher risk of having twins. The genetic factors seem to be completely independent, however: women with DZ twins in the family give birth to more twins of the DZ sort, while those with MZ twins in the family have more MZ twins.

A woman who bears twins is often older. Most twins are born to women aged 25–34, but the likelihood of twins in any one pregnancy is higher in women 35–40, because this is when a double ovulation is most likely. It seems that twins in this age bracket will probably rise as more and more babies are born to women in their 40s. Many women now put off starting their family until their late thirties and, while the birth rate among twenty-somethings has dropped, the number of babies born to women in their forties has gone up by over 50 per cent in ten years.

The older mother does not always welcome the arrival of twins. Her own relatives may be elderly, so she is less likely to have the benefit of an extended family, and she could face health problems of her own. She may even find herself sandwiched in a generation of women who have to care for ailing relatives while simultaneously bringing up their own children. On the other hand, the older mother is often more mature, socially stable, more highly educated and in a better financial position to bring up two babies.

Because of her age and fertility, a woman pregnant with twins may have several children already (she is what doctors call multiparous). She is often taller than average too. This probably reflects good nutrition rather than anything else – healthy women are more likely to carry two or more babies to a viable age. In the animal kingdom, the reverse applies – smaller mammals tend to produce most multiples – undoubtedly because small animals are preyed on and therefore have to have larger litters if the species is to survive.

Whatever her age or height, a mother of twins is on average more fertile. According to figures from Canada, Scotland, Denmark and elsewhere, there was a peak in twin births nine months after the end of World War II. The peak in twin births actually came two or three months earlier than the post-war baby boom as a whole, suggesting that these women may have found it especially easy to conceive.

Unfortunately, not all women expecting twins had intended to conceive at all, let alone to end up with the patter of two pairs of tiny feet. In one of her research projects, TAMBA's midwifery advisor Jane Spillman found that on average some 16 per cent of mothers of twins questioned had not planned on becoming pregnant yet. Many of these were using contraception, but it had failed them.

Studies have suggested that mothers of twins are more fertile because, on the whole, they have fewer period problems than most women and their pituitary glands secrete higher levels of follicle-stimulating hormone (FSH), which could be why they are more likely to produce two eggs in any one cycle. FSH levels rise with increasing years and this may help explain why age is a risk factor in twinning.

One interesting theory about the high twinning rate in the Yoruba tribe concerns yams, which are an important part of the diet in rural Nigeria and may exert a hormone-like effect. Yoruba women who migrate to the big city and adopt a more urban diet tend to leave behind their amazingly high rate of twinning. However, it is not certain that food is the cause.

Incidentally, the hormone status of women who have twins may have other interesting consequences. Although it is far from proven yet, studies suggest that women who have twins might run a lower risk of breast cancer.

· *What Will Your Twins Be Like?* ·

Will your twins be identical or not? There is an approximate chance of two in three that they will be non-identical (DZ) and if they are of different sexes this will clinch it: by definition boy–girl pairs cannot be identical. If they are the same sex, there are a number of helpful clues to look for, though others are misleading.

Many people, including some obstetricians and midwives, still believe that the presence of two placentas means that the twins are non-identical, while one means they are identical. However, this is not always true, as the diagram on page 21 shows.

In non-identicals (DZ), about half the twin pairs have a fused placenta while the rest have two separate placentas. Identicals (MZ) are more likely to have a fused placenta, but they too can have separate placentas. Only in identicals can there be just one chorionic membrane separating the babies. Therefore, if the membranes are carefully examined after delivery and there's only one chorion, the twins must be identical. (Your hospital may be able to do this for you – ask in advance.)

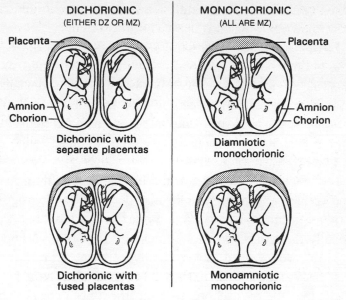

Types of twins and their placentas

What happens in an MZ-twin pregnancy depends on when the fertilized ovum, or zygote, divides into two.

- If division happens within three days of fertilization, the twins are dichorionic.
- If it is between three and nine days after fertilization, they will be monochorionic but diamniotic. In other words, there will still be two separate sacs in the womb.
- If division takes place between nine and twelve days after fertilization, the twins will be monochorionic and monoamniotic (sharing the same sac).
- If it is after twelve days (some experts say fifteen days) the twins could be conjoined.

Siamese (conjoined) twins

Some women worry about the possibility of producing Siamese twins, so called because the original pair of conjoined twins, Chang and Eng, born in 1811, came from Siam (now known as Thailand).

Births of Siamese twins are reported in the media from time to time, but they are really very rare. On average, there is perhaps one case in every 50 000 to 100 000 pregnancies. Such cases are usually picked up by ultrasound scan during pregnancy, often because the babies seem to be lying in a strange position. Occasionally, though, conjoined twins are diagnosed only during labour.

For some reason, they are more often female than male. The connection between them may be small and insignificant, for instance just a band of tissue at chest level, but occasionally the connection may be more difficult or even impossible to sever without losing one of the twins. In rare cases they may share one or more vital organs, such as a heart. Sometimes the connections between them are extensive but still compatible with life, in which case the twins are often able to lead fairly fulfilled lives, including marriage and children. Understandably, compromise between the twins is essential.

· *How Identical are 'Identicals'?* ·

So-called identical twins are often described as being like two peas in a pod, but they are not necessarily identical. If you look closely, there are always some differences, for instance in their freckles or the shape of the head.

> Although my girls are officially identical I've always been able to tell them apart, except in photos taken as tiny babies when I can't remember who wore what! Rachel and Zoe just look and sound different to me and even feel different. If one of them pads into the bedroom in the night for a hug, I can always tell who it is!

Nobody knows for sure why identicals are not always identical. It is likely that there are different reasons which apply to different sets of twins, such as:

- differences in birth weight
- differences in blood flow in the womb
- differences in position in the womb
- birth order (hence different experiences in labour)
- mirror-imaging
- chromosome inactivation.

Mirror-imaging is a harmless but fascinating phenomenon which probably affects a quarter of identical twins. In mirror-image twins, hair patterns, handedness and fingerprints can be reversed, literally as if seen in a mirror. This is not necessarily linked with any internal disorders, such as situs inversus, in which major organs are shifted from left to right and vice versa. In fact, it usually causes no problems at all, except for the rather obvious fact that if a left-handed child sits on the right of a right-handed child at a table, neither of them can write, draw or eat very easily. About 35 per cent of MZ twins are left-handed, double the rate in the general population, so it is an important practical point. The cause of mirror-imaging isn't known, but it seems to be one of those things that catches the public's imagination.

Chromosome inactivation refers to the fact that, although identicals have the same chromosomes, sometimes one in effect lies dormant, which explains why even some inherited conditions, like muscular dystrophy, do not affect both 'identical' twins.

Zygosity – Identical or not?

If you have a same-sex pair, they may be very alike, just like two sisters or brothers can be. You can get a good idea of whether or not they are identical by looking carefully at certain features. Identical twins can differ in weight, height and shape of head, but they have the same

- hair colour
- eye colour
- skin colour
- blood group.

So, if twins are dissimilar in any of these respects, they are not identical. The shape of the ears is said to be quite a useful indicator, as it is less likely to be affected by position in the womb than is the head shape as a whole; ears, therefore, tend to look the same in identicals.

Fairly simple laboratory tests – looking at the placenta and membranes and checking blood groups – are up to 80 per cent accurate in determining identicalness (or zygosity, as it is scientifically known). So how can one tell for sure?

DNA fingerprinting

DNA (deoxyribonucleic acid) carries the genetic code and is sometimes referred to as the building block of life. DNA fingerprinting is a way of testing for many different DNA characteristics at the same time. Identical (MZ) twins have the same DNA fingerprints, while non-identical (DZ) twins have one chance in about one in 3×10^{14} of being the same; that's a probability of one in 300 000 000 000 000, so you can consider the test to be pretty conclusive. However, it is likely to give completely misleading results if done within a few months of a blood transfusion.

DNA fingerprinting is a technique used in forensic science and may be done on the hair, skin and semen of suspects. It can also be done on the placenta or a small amount of cord blood of babies, and even on a stillborn baby.

The test is expensive and at present no agency can guarantee to pay for it, so the cost may fall on you. If you are not sure whether you want it carried out, you could ask if the hospital could freeze some cord blood for later. If your twins have already been born, paediatricians advise parents to think carefully about the wisdom of subjecting them to blood tests before they start clamouring for DNA fingerprinting.

Does it matter if your twins are identical? It may be important if you are contemplating another pregnancy, since you are slightly more likely to have a second set of twins if the first set was DZ. Most parents like to know anyway, even if their family is complete. A study done for the Multiple Births Foundation (MBF) confirms that most mothers do consider it important, yet, of the mothers interviewed, over half had been given inaccurate information, based on incorrect assumptions about the placenta and zygosity. They would have done better had they simply taken a wild guess!

> I don't know if my boys are identical or not. I don't really mind one way or the other. But people do ask and I feel stupid not being able to give an accurate answer. Besides, my sons have started to ask if they came from the same egg.

· *Twins and Growth* ·

Interestingly, there tends to be a greater discrepancy in birth weight between identical twins than non-identical twins, probably because in the womb the former sometimes share their blood flow, though unequally.

Even when there are marked differences in weight or height, in the case of identicals these usually even up as the years pass. Non-identicals tend to differ more as they grow up and there is no more reason for them to be the same size than there is for any other two siblings. It is just that when children are exactly the same age the differences are most obvious. Same-sex pairs are usually more alike as adults than are boy–girl pairs.

Twins generally grow just as tall as singletons, though studies show that they are often a bit thinner. Both MZ and DZ twins are below the average weight for the population but are of average height. Paediatrician Dr John Buckler, an expert in the growth of multiples, points out that this may mean that in adulthood the twins will be somewhat shorter than their parents; as mentioned earlier, parents of twins tend to be taller than average. For the same reason, twins are often smaller in stature than their non-twin siblings too.

Girl twins, for some mysterious reason, often achieve comparatively greater height than boys, but even so the boy will, as a man, be on average 13 cm taller than his twin sister. The growth of triplets is believed to be similar to that of twins, but much less information is available here. Buckler plans to carry out longitudinal studies (i.e., looking at the same sample of children over a long period of time) to find out more about the growth of twins.

· *Intelligence* ·

It is sometimes said that twins are not as bright as singletons and many studies do show that IQ (intelligence quotient), as measured in formal tests, tends to be a few points lower in twins. However, a few points rarely matter in everyday life – or even in academic life – and these average findings can tell you nothing about your own twins, either (or both) of whom may be very bright. There is no evidence of any significant difference between twins and singletons in intelligence. Nor should you assume, if you have other children, that they will be brighter than your twins.

Twins can, however, differ from each other. One of the longest-running longitudinal studies is the ongoing Louisville Twin Study in Kentucky. It began over 30 years ago and looked at both the physical and mental development of twins.

Work from Louisville and elsewhere suggests that, as with height and weight, MZ twins tend to be similar in IQ while DZ pairs become less alike as the years go by.

One interesting finding is that the IQ of boy–girl pairs is more similar than that of same-sex DZ pairs. But why? Perhaps because same-sex pairs need to go to great lengths to express their individuality, while boy–girl pairs don't have to: the differences between them are obvious enough not to need emphasizing by behaving in dissimilar ways.

This brings me to the interplay between genetics and the environment, something which is at the heart of the debate about nature versus nurture in general and the study of twins in particular. Take reading, for instance. Researchers at the Institute of Child Health, London, studying language problems in twins – a topic explored in Chapter 9 – have confirmed that identicals tend to have similar delays, whereas non-identicals do not. Part of the explanation may lie in the fact that identicals are more often treated as one unit, although this is certainly not the only reason. For example, a mother may be more likely to read to her children together, or to address them simultaneously, if they look very alike.

A great deal of work is being undertaken in these and other areas. One organization responsible for bringing together all kinds of scientists in the field of twin work is the International Society for Twin Studies, formed in 1974 by the geneticist Professor Luigi Gedda and based, appropriately enough, in Rome, the city supposedly founded by Romulus.

· *Triplets and more* ·

What if you are having triplets or an even higher multiple? First of all, if you are expecting three or more babies, you are slightly more likely to have more girls than boys. The more babies you produce at once, the higher will be the proportion of girls. About 51 per cent of all single-born babies – but only 46 per cent of quadruplets – are male.

Like twins, triplets can arise in more than one way. They are often trizygotic – developing from three fertilized ova. Sometimes they are dizygotic (from two ova, one of which splits to form a monozygotic pair which are then identical). On rare occasions, they can be monozygotic (one fertilized egg splits and one of those halves splits again).

Much the same applies – though in a more complicated way – to higher-order births. The Dionne quintuplets, born in Canada in the 1930s, are believed to be identical (MZ).

> Whenever I was out with my three (two girls and a boy), I'd be asked how they were conceived. I thought they were ignorant, and wondered if I was supposed to draw them a picture. But then of course I realized that they wanted to know if they were test tube babies or all our own work.

· *Infertility Treatment and* ·
Multiple Births

Only a third, or even less, of triplet and higher-order births are conceived in the old-fashioned way, the rest being due to various forms of infertility treatment. This helps explain the phenomenal rise in triplets in the last decade.

Assisted-conception techniques raise all sorts of complex ethical questions, many of which – like the fate of frozen embryos – are outside the scope of this book. Looking simply at the practical issues, it is obvious that large numbers of multiple births, together with the medical advances which enable more tiny babies to survive, put huge pressure on hospital services.

As one obstetrician in training put it:

A few years back, I was going around the Special Care Baby Unit early one morning, when I realized that it was literally full of triplets. In terms of our methods in the infertility clinic, I began to think of multiple pregnancy less as a success and more as a disaster.

Fertility problems are said to affect one couple in every six, increasing numbers of whom seek help for their difficulties in conceiving. Worldwide, various assisted reproduction techniques are responsible for a 20 to 33 per cent risk of twins or more.

At first sight, *in vitro* fertilization (IVF) is the most obvious culprit. In this technique, the woman is made to superovulate with drugs to produce as many eggs (ova) as possible. Her eggs are then collected, fertilized in the laboratory and then replaced as embryos into the womb.

To maximize the chances of success, more than one embryo is implanted, but how many is the right number? Too few and the technique will fail. Too many and very high-order pregnancies can result, with an increased risk of losing one or more embryos (and therefore of failure).

Infertility units are becoming more responsible and increasingly aware that replacing fewer embryos can actually result in a better success rate, if you consider the end-point that really matters to prospective parents – not the raw figures for numbers of pregnancies achieved by a clinic offering IVF, but the take-home baby rate.

Incidentally, IVF produces multiples from different ova, at least in theory. In practice, it sometimes results in multiples which are identical (MZ) too, which means that triplets, say, from IVF are not always trizygotic. Fertility specialists now believe that something changes in the outer layer (called the zona pellucida) of the ovum during the process of IVF, so that the covering becomes more brittle and thus more likely to divide to produce two identical embryos.

In Britain, no more than three embryos are replaced in IVF. This guidance was introduced in the 1991 HFEA (Human Fertilization and Embryology Authority) Code of Practice. The situation in other countries varies. In Ireland, until recently all embryos produced had to be transferred back into the womb. In France, there is no control over the number of embryos, but fewer are being replaced than before. Embryo reduction (described in the Appendix) is also actively promoted there.

IVF may now be the best-regulated fertility technique in Britain, but it is not the only one. There is also GIFT (gamete intra-fallopian transfer), for example, as well as the much more common methods of inducing ovulation. These are not always used appropriately or in a controlled way.

In fact, many more triplets now result from ovulation induction rather than IVF in the UK, a point which some doctors have yet to acknowledge. The National Study of Triplet and Higher Order Births in 1990 found that 35 per cent of mothers with triplets had had ovulation induction, as had 70 per cent of mothers with quadruplets.

Drugs which bring on ovulation are a relatively low-tech treatment for infertility and are easy to give, but they can cause problems if given without proper monitoring. A woman may not know, until it's too late, that she has produced two, three, or even more eggs in one cycle instead of the required one.

> I resented it deeply. Yes, I got pregnant when I wanted, but all I asked for was one baby at a time.

Some GPs and a few hospital doctors are prescribing ovulation-inducing drugs in this way. Although it is a much quicker way of achieving a pregnancy than waiting for an appointment at a specialist clinic, it is becoming clear that inducing ovulation with drugs can do women a disservice unless carefully monitored.

Couples undergoing treatment for fertility problems should be told of the risk of multiple pregnancy. The HFEA even makes it obligatory for every centre performing IVF to offer counselling, so that would-be parents do know they could have twins, triplets, or more. However, there is a big difference between hearing what is said and absorbing all the practical implications.

A couple may be so desperate for a child that multiple pregnancy seems a small price to pay and they are likely to underestimate the risk as well as the problems. Older women especially may feel that time is running out. Others may even welcome the thought of an instant family, particularly if they are making huge sacrifices to fund their treatment, as many do when unable to obtain it on the NHS.

Quite apart from the cost of the treatment itself, bringing up babies is expensive. In 1996 a report from the supermarket group Asda estimated that one infant's first year could set parents back by as much as £2500 and £6000. For equipment alone, one baby can cost something like £1000 if you buy clothing, bedding and so on from scratch. Since you need to duplicate almost everything (except for obvious items like baby baths) for each baby born at the same time, triplets could cost nearly £3000. Then there is the possible loss of one parent's income, if only temporarily, and often a simultaneous need for a larger home. Many families with multiples are forced to consider building an extension or taking on a larger mortgage at a time when finances are particularly tight.

Very small babies often have a struggle to survive. Setting aside the potential impact on a family's emotional and financial resources if one or more babies is disabled and needs extra provision, even healthy multiples exact a high manpower cost. It has been estimated by a mother of triplets that babycare and related household chores eat up 197.5 hours per week, a schedule that would stagger even a junior hospital doctor. Since there are only 168 hours in a week, extra help has to be enlisted (and funded), or many tasks must be dropped altogether.

It is not easy going through assisted-fertility treatment and when it produces multiples a couple can have a hard time acknowledging the difficulties they face. This is the hoped-for parenthood – to whom can they admit their doubts? Can they own up to not being perfect? People are not always sympathetic and may even tell a couple that they have brought their troubles on themselves. TAMBA runs an Infertility Support Group which can help parents deal with these and other issues, as well as Supertwins and Special Needs groups.

Chapter Two

YOUR MULTIPLE PREGNANCY

Being pregnant with two or more babies often feels different from being pregnant with one, if only on grounds of size. Until about 28 to 32 weeks into the pregnancy, the growth of each twin (and possibly each triplet) is roughly the same as that of a single baby. This means that at any one stage of pregnancy you will be much bulkier. For instance, at 20 weeks, the fundus (the top end) of the womb can be felt at 20 cm (8 inches) above the pubic bone in a singleton pregnancy, but, if you're expecting twins, your fundus is likely to be higher by 4 cm (1^1/2 inches) or more. By the time you get to 28 weeks, you could be looking and feeling as large as a woman carrying one baby at term.

By the time you get to term, the volume of your womb could be nearly twice as big. Scientific studies show that at term the inner volume of the uterus is 5 litres (about 9 pints) with singletons and nearly 10 litres (17^1/2 pints) with twins!

> I was vast. Something poked under my ribs constantly from about 30 weeks and the side view in the mirror was alarming – I've kept photos to prove it. By 37 weeks I could hardly sit with my legs together because the bump took so much room.

Fortunately, you probably won't be pregnant for quite as long as with a singleton.

- While 40 weeks is 'full term' for a single baby, 37 weeks is considered to be full term for twins, with identicals often arriving slightly earlier than non-identicals.

- For triplets, the average length of gestation is 34 weeks.
- For quads, it is 33 weeks – nearly two months shorter than a singleton pregnancy.

Premature labour, when the babies arrive earlier than anticipated, is one of the main hazards of twin and higher-order pregnancies. This is dealt with in Chapter 3. Other symptoms and complications which can be commoner in multiple pregnancy are covered here, along with the important physical and emotional adjustments you need to make before your babies arrive.

Twice as pregnant?

A few women carrying multiples just know, in some cases long before their first scan, that they are carrying more than one baby. You may need to wear your maternity dresses a lot earlier than you expected (although this is quite common in second and subsequent pregnancies anyway, perhaps because a woman's abdominal muscles are weaker by then). Or you may notice that you are a slightly different shape, with a small but definite bulge towards the sides rather than just at the front. You may also feel more kicks than you might have anticipated. Some women have enjoyed getting the better of their professionals:

I just knew something was different and soon after I had the pregnancy test I started wondering aloud whether I was having twins. I was feeling a lot sicker than with my first one, though a doctor friend of mine said I was probably just having a girl this time. The junior doctor in the clinic didn't believe me either. She sent me for a scan, having written on the form 'to exclude twins'. I left the clinic thinking, 'What rubbish – surely she means "to confirm twins".'

Before the scan confirmed twins, I was grilled by the midwife in the clinic who thought my pregnancy was simply more advanced than I was admitting. She asked me several times if I was sure of my 'dates', i.e. of my last period, which I was. In fact, as an accountant, I was somewhat insulted by her apparent accusation and I retorted huffily that I knew not only the days of the week but also the months of the year.

· *Weight Changes* ·

Weight gain in pregnancy varies, not just according to how well your babies are growing, but also on whether you were overweight to start with. Some women put on almost 25 kg (4 stone) while carrying twins, though most gain less than this. How much *you* should gain – and when – is hard to say, especially with quads and other higher-order births because there just are not that many of them born to work out a useful guide. However, a number of studies taken together suggest that a good or 'recommended' weight gain would be:

- For a twin pregnancy, a total gain of 18 kg (40 lb), preferably 11 kg (24 lb) by week 24, and then 0.6 kg ($1^1/4$ lb) a week until birth.
- For triplets, a total gain of 22.7 kg (50 lb), preferably 16 kg (36 lb) by week 24, then 0.6 kg ($1^1/4$ lb) a week until birth.
- For quads, a total gain of 31 kg (68 lb).

· *Other Bodily Changes* ·

Along with increasing bulk go a number of inner changes. The way a woman's body adapts to carrying and nourishing more than one fetus at a time has not been nearly as well studied as the average singleton pregnancy, but there are a few known changes.

Heart and circulation

In the mother's circulation, the volume of blood (or to be exact the volume of plasma, which is the blood minus all the cells carried in it) begins to expand in the first three months of pregnancy. It rises rapidly in the second three months and continues to increase, although more slowly, to reach a plateau a few weeks before birth. So, if you are carrying just one baby, your final maximum blood volume in pregnancy is nearly 50 per cent greater than it was before you were pregnant. In a twin pregnancy, however, the staggering fact is that its maximum is nearly double your pre-pregnant level (not that you will notice it – the increase is all inside the blood vessels).

To cope with the increase in blood volume and pump it around the bloodstream, your heart will have to work a lot harder in a multiple pregnancy. This won't matter much unless you already happen to have some heart trouble, or plan to undertake strenuous exercise in late pregnancy. In practical terms, this means you should not play squash, for instance, towards the end of your twin pregnancy, although you probably won't feel like it anyway. If you have any queries as to how much sport you can or cannot play, check with your doctor.

Anaemia

Carrying more than one baby uses up a mother's reserves of both iron and folic acid. It is estimated that a pregnant woman needs an extra 570 mg of iron for herself during pregnancy, plus around 430 mg for each fetus. In fact, a woman's stores of iron are often low in a multiple pregnancy, though this will not show up unless you have some complicated test, like a bone-marrow examination, which is not done routinely.

A woman who is well nourished herself can often handle the extra demands of twin pregnancy without becoming anaemic and research from Scotland shows that anaemia is not much more common in twin pregnancy. For this reason, obstetricians nowadays tend not to give mothers iron tablets routinely in pregnancy, whether you are having twins or not. However, many GPs and midwives still do so automatically.

Obviously, if you were to develop anaemia, you would need treatment (usually with tablets, but sometimes by injection). Anaemia is one of the conditions which show up on routine antenatal blood tests and you may have been told, or seen from the records, your Hb (haemoglobin) level. However, Hb should not be taken at face value: it is normal for it to drop, but this is because the blood volume expands, as explained above. After 20 weeks, for instance, the average Hb in a twin pregnancy is around 10 g/dl (the normal Hb level is 12 to 14), not necessarily because the woman is getting dangerously anaemic but because the red blood cells are swimming in a larger volume. It is one of the other figures in the blood result (the average Hb concentration *per cell*) that shows whether true anaemia is present.

· *Symptoms of Pregnancy* ·

Many women feel at their best in pregnancy, while others find this supposedly joyous time marred by one or more symptoms, such as:

- nausea or vomiting
- heartburn
- constipation
- headache
- varicose veins
- piles
- backache
- sleeplessness.

In practice these can be quite troublesome, yet they are still considered minor problems (and often dismissed by doctors) because they are not medically serious. They are caused mainly by the sheer size of the enlarging uterus, the hormones of pregnancy, or the way your body is having to adapt. In some cases, the worse the symptoms, the better the babies are growing, so no wonder medics can remain unimpressed by your complaints. There are tips on how to care for yourself and cope with pregnancy symptoms later in this chapter.

· *Medical Complications* ·

Aches and pains apart, multiple pregnancy tends to be more complicated from the purely medical angle. The possibility of complications, however remote it may seem to you, is one very good reason for antenatal care. During a multiple pregnancy the doctor or midwife may want to keep a closer eye on you than if you were having only one baby.

A twin or higher-order pregnancy is not the norm for humans, something mothers-to-be (and those caring for them) need to remember. The extra risk involved in a twin pregnancy is a fact you just have to accept, regardless of how easy or straightforward any previous pregnancy may have been. While there is no need to lie awake worrying about rare disorders, don't get too blasé either.

This should be a happy and enjoyable time for you. In many cases you can still have shared care (antenatal care provided jointly by hospital staff and by community staff) and carry on seeing the midwife, but you may need to attend a little more often and have more frequent scans. You may also find that you see more people at each visit, not just because twins are more interesting to professionals but because teamwork is an important ingredient of effective antenatal care and a good way of ensuring the best outcome for you and your babies.

Although most women sail through their multiple pregnancy without any of the following complications, statistically there is a risk of:

- vaginal bleeding (including miscarriage, placental abruption and antepartum haemorrhage)
- pre-eclampsia (toxaemia) (see page 40)
- growth retardation of the fetus(es)
- hydramnios (see page 41)
- twin-to-twin transfusion syndrome (see Appendix, page 320).

I must apologize if any readers are put off or even alarmed by the explanations below. You can skip them if you don't want to read them. However, like many other doctors, I believe that being aware of the possibilities is to be forearmed and could, in my opinion, save your babies' lives.

Vaginal bleeding

This is said to be nearly three times more common in twin than single pregnancy, though precise figures are hard to come by. The exact cause of the increased risk is unknown. One might expect a higher incidence of placenta praevia (where one or other placenta lies very low in the womb) purely because in a multiple pregnancy more of the uterus is taken up by placentas, but this doesn't wholly explain the extra risk of bleeding in twin or higher-order pregnancies.

Bleeding in pregnancy actually comes from the wall of the womb, not from the babies. All the same, the heavier the blood loss, the more likely it is to be serious, as you might guess. Many women who bleed in pregnancy will deliver normal babies, but this should not be assumed. Always contact your doctor or midwife without delay if you bleed while pregnant.

Pre-eclampsia

Not all pregnant women have heard of pre-eclampsia (also known as toxaemia of pregnancy, or PET), yet it is the commonest cause of maternal death in Britain and it can also kill one or both babies, so it is clearly worth taking seriously.

PET is commoner in primigravidae (first-time mothers) and is thought to be caused by some abnormality of the placenta, or placentas. It is not clear quite what the problem is and research is under way in order that PET may be better understood and treated.

PET affects the growth of the fetus and causes raised blood pressure, protein in the mother's urine and fluid retention. An early symptom is often excess weight gain, for instance, more than 1 kg (just over 2 lb) in a week. Picking up PET early is one of the most important reasons for keeping antenatal appointments. Blood pressure, urine and weight should be checked each time (though the last measurement seems to be going out of favour). Along with many other doctors, I believe PET is a compelling argument against further cuts in antenatal care.

PET is more common in twin pregnancies. Mild forms of PET affect about a fifth of all first-time mothers expecting singletons and about a quarter of those expecting twins. Serious PET, where protein is present in the urine, is about half as common as this. If severe, PET can cause eclampsia in the woman. Typically, she will suffer from fits (convulsions) and sometimes lasting kidney damage.

If PET is diagnosed, the priority is usually to deliver the baby or babies, assuming they are mature enough to survive happily outside the womb. Deciding when to deliver is a little more difficult with multiples than it is with singletons. Sometimes treating raised blood pressure in its own right can help treat PET.

Hydramnios

Hydramnios (also called polyhydramnios) is excess amniotic fluid, often to the point where it becomes uncomfortable for the woman, as well as being more difficult for the midwife to feel the fetus.

Hydramnios affects around 5 per cent of multiple pregnancies. Draining off some of the fluid can make the mother more comfortable. On the other hand, there is some risk that this will trigger premature labour. The real importance of hydramnios is that it can be linked with other complications, in particular twin-to-twin transfusion syndrome. Therefore, if you seem to have too much amniotic fluid, you will probably be sent for another ultrasound scan to make sure everything is all right.

· *Ultrasound Scans* ·

Ultrasound scans (USS) use waves of the same type as sound. When they first came in, it was assumed that they were completely safe because they use no X-rays, but in the last few years, one or two doubts have been raised about both the increasing role and the ultimate safety of USS. Conclusive answers are not available, but ultrasound has been in wide use since the 1970s and has not yet been proven to be harmful in any way.

USS has many uses, such as:

- confirming the expected date of delivery
- locating the placenta (for instance, diagnosing placenta praevia)
- picking up congenital abnormalities
- enabling tests like amniocentesis and chorionic villus sampling (CVS) to be done safely
- identifying breech babies before labour (this can affect the method of delivery).

In multiple pregnancies, USS plays an important additional role in:

- detecting twin and higher-order pregnancies in the first place
- monitoring the growth of each baby
- picking up abnormalities in cases where blood tests cannot help
- detecting which twin pregnancies are at especially high risk (see the section on chorionicity in the Appendix)
- diagnosing complications of pregnancy, such as twin-to-twin transfusion syndrome (again, see the Appendix)
- observing the interaction of twins before birth (see Chapter 8).

Diagnosing multiples

Your first contact with the USS department may well be momentous, since this is probably when you will discover (officially) that you are expecting more than one baby. Actually, all first scans carried out in pregnancy should check for twins because not every woman has symptoms or a family tree suggesting that she is likely to have multiples. Usually the first scan is at around eighteen weeks, but may be much earlier if, for instance:

- you have fertility treatment
- you are unsure of the date of your last period
- you have symptoms such as bleeding.

Many departments can pick up twins and more with 95 to 100 per cent accuracy, so the days when over half of all twins came as a surprise in the delivery suite are, thankfully, long gone. But twins can still be missed if a scan is done very early (much before 12 weeks), especially with an inexperienced sonographer, as the USS technician is called.

Occasionally triplets have been misdiagnosed. About 6 per cent of triplets and 16 per cent of quads are not spotted until scans later in pregnancy. It is unusual, though not unknown, for the news 'It's twins' to be upgraded to 'It's triplets' on the next scan and even to quads on a subsequent scan . . . . At least you will be lying down if and when you hear this; it is said that one cannot faint while horizontal.

For most women, the exciting fact that they're having twins comes as a huge shock. The way in which the news is presented can add to the distress:

> The technician just frowned at the screen and muttered darkly under her breath. She didn't seem to hear me when I asked if everything was OK. She only said that she'd have to get a colleague in and wouldn't be long. I lay there and my life flashed before me. My baby was deformed. The news just cut everything in two: before and after. I was in shock. The technician came back with someone else after what seemed like ages and then I was told I was having twins. It was such a relief but I could hardly believe it.

It may seem unreal to begin with and while you are on your way home you may begin to doubt whether you heard right. Many USS departments can, for a small fee, give you a photo of the scan to keep. It is said that this can help get you used to the idea of two (or more) babies, but, whether you have a picture or not, your first scan is likely to be the moment that begins your lifelong relationship with your children.

It would be nice if staff could help answer queries about twins soon after the scan, but often this is not possible. However, just after you leave the USS department is a good time to get in touch with TAMBA if you haven't already; many women are greatly helped by being given the number for their local twins' club or for the TAMBA Twinline by the hospital staff directly after their scan confirms twins.

Monitoring growth

Other things being equal, the larger the bump, the better the baby is growing, but in a twin pregnancy what can the overall size tell you about each baby? Not much.

A woman expecting twins is therefore usually scanned regularly from 28 weeks, perhaps at fortnightly intervals. This is the time when the growth of twins can fall off slightly, so scans in the later part of pregnancy check on the growth of each baby separately. They also play an important part in diagnosing twin-to-twin transfusion syndrome.

Early pregnancy loss

It is a sad fact of life that occasionally both babies do not survive the full span of the pregnancy. Some women who have early scans showing twins will lose one of the fetuses long before term, either with or without vaginal bleeding. Occasionally the symptoms are typical of a miscarriage, but the woman goes on feeling pregnant and her pregnancy test stays positive, because one fetus of a twin pregnancy has miscarried, not the whole pregnancy.

Although one cannot predict which women will be affected, the risk of early pregnancy loss is higher before twelve weeks and highest of all before eight weeks. It follows that the earlier you have a scan, the more often this phenomenon is seen. The so-called 'vanishing twin' syndrome is something about which little was known before scanning became routine, but now it is becoming clear that it may be quite common.

There is a very high rate of early pregnancy loss with singletons too. In fact, the more one learns, the more likely it appears that many pregnancies come to grief. Unfair as it may seem, we don't know why this happens. Some experts believe that perhaps only a quarter of natural pregnancies reach full term and that 12 to 15 per cent of all live births may start off as twins.

The outlook for the surviving baby seems to be excellent. However, if you lose one of your babies, you and your partner may have feelings you need to express in order to come to terms with the experience.

Picking up abnormalities

In many hospitals, a so-called anomaly scan is offered, usually at twenty weeks, though it can be done much earlier, at ten to fourteen weeks. Often it is done only if:

- there is a family history or previous history of some genetic defect
- the mother is diabetic
- hydramnios has been diagnosed.

If you are not offered one of these scans, you may be able to request one, but you may have to pay.

An anomaly scan in twins takes twice as long as in singleton pregnancies. It can pick up various abnormalities, for instance, in the heart, stomach, abdominal wall and the spine or central nervous system. However, spotting that something's amiss is often only the first stage in diagnosing the problem; you may need further tests. If your obstetrician is going to suggest any major intervention on the basis of USS findings, the scan will probably need to be repeated to make sure any action is based on the most accurate and up-to-date information.

Nuchal translucency

This refers to whether or not there's a 'space', or rather a translucency filled with fluid, behind the neck of a fetus on an USS. This can be an early sign of Down's syndrome (trisomy

21) and sometimes of other disorders too, especially heart abnormalities.

It is a particularly useful sign in multiple pregnancy because so far no other effective means has been discovered of screening for Down's syndrome in twin and higher-order pregnancies. The test is offered in many centres and looks likely to become routine. It is done at between eleven and thirteen weeks, usually through the mother's abdomen, like any other USS, but to get a good picture sometimes the probe has to be placed in the vagina.

Remember that nuchal translucency is just a screening method, not the final diagnosis. If you have a positive nuchal translucency, you will be offered a further test (CVS or amniocentesis) to get a definite answer. In most cases, the results of these so-called invasive tests will still be normal, but you will be given the chance to have an anomaly scan later on anyway. In the unlikely event of an abnormality being confirmed, couples will get further advice from the hospital.

· *Antenatal Screening* ·

Having tests, and waiting for results, is worrying. On the other hand, many women find tests reassuring. There is a lot of confusion as to what antenatal tests can and cannot do and there are special problems in multiple pregnancy, so let's consider the issue as a whole.

A growing part of antenatal care is devoted to screening for a range of fetal disorders, particularly Down's syndrome and neural tube defects (NTD). NTD is the term medics give to a spectrum of central nervous system abnormalities, the best known being spina bifida and anencephaly (under-development of the whole skull). Tests can be:

- invasive (e.g. amniocentesis or CVS)
- non-invasive (e.g. USS or taking blood from the mother).

Screening in a twin or higher-order pregnancy can be difficult technically; for instance in interpreting the result (of non-invasive tests), or because even more expertise is needed to do an invasive test safely. Then, on the ethical and emotional side, what can one do about the result? If you have objections to termination under any circumstances, there is little point in having some of these antenatal tests. You will have your own view.

Twin pregnancies where only one baby is affected present a further dilemma. It is now possible in some circumstances selectively to terminate a multiple pregnancy (this topic is covered in the Appendix), a decision which is a huge responsibility for any couple facing this situation. It is bad enough to lose and grieve for a singleton, but psychologists have found that mourning for one baby while simultaneously caring for another of the same age can create conflict. On the other hand, multiples can be challenging enough to parent when healthy, let alone when one of them is severely disabled.

Then there are the general cautions which ought to be (but are not always) given with all antenatal screening. Tests do not necessarily give 100 per cent positive or negative results and they can occasionally mislead. Some tests only give the probability of a baby being affected and the figures are not always easy to understand. If the result is greater than one in 300 (say it's one in 150), the test is usually said to be positive. If the result is smaller than one in 300 (say one in 400), it's said to be negative (yes, that is the right way round).

An added complication is that, while the result may give the likely diagnosis, it may not say much about how severely affected this particular baby is likely to be. As an example, anencephaly is fairly straightforward because it's usually lethal, but a child who has Down's syndrome can be very happy and affectionate, and fulfilling to parent. Need I point out that not every so-called normal child is all of those things?

All this may sound depressing, but pregnant women and the professionals caring for them should consider these issues in advance, not after a positive result is received. In fact, a negative result is far and away the likeliest outcome and it can be very reassuring. Here too a note of caution should be added: screening doesn't tell you everything is OK. In the last analysis, life and creating life are still something of a gamble. There is no such thing as a guarantee of a perfect baby.

You won't need much luck: over 98 per cent of babies over- all are born completely healthy, so the chances are that you won't have to confront any of these dilemmas. However, it is important to know, before you have any tests, the route you could be travelling down. Your obstetrician, GP or midwife can certainly help you make your decisions, though ultimately you and your partner have to make up your own minds.

Your worries

With twins or higher multiples, you may be more worried than with a singleton pregnancy. After all, are not two or more healthy babies a lot to ask for? But in fact abnormalities are not that much more common with multiples than with single babies. Down's syndrome, for instance, is no more like- ly, as long as you allow for the fact that mothers of twins tend to be slightly older. A few identical twins seem to run a slightly higher risk of some conditions, mostly abnormalities of the midline body organs, but these are really rarities. Cerebral palsy is estimated to be more common in multiples, but this may have to do with the fact that more small vulner- able babies are surviving.

Anxiety is probably an integral part of pregnancy and

indeed of parenting. It has been said that it would be almost noteworthy to find an expectant mother who didn't worry about the health of her unborn babies. Of course, if anxiety begins to take over and interfere with your ability to enjoy life or to look forward to the future, you need to talk things over with someone you trust, like your midwife or doctor.

· *Non-Invasive Tests* ·

Nuchal translucency and anomaly scans were both covered earlier, in the section on ultrasound scans. The other common non-invasive tests are AFP and the so-called triple test.

Alphafetoprotein (AFP)

This is a blood test that you can have at around sixteen weeks of pregnancy; it tests for spina bifida and other NTDs. AFP is a protein made by the baby's liver and a certain amount spills over into the mother's bloodstream (hence its usefulness). A high AFP level may indicate a higher risk of spina bifida and NTDs, but twinning also causes an elevated AFP level. So, whilst a very high level can be helpful, on the whole AFP levels are misleading with multiples and of course tell you nothing about the health of each individual baby.

Some women happen to have an AFP test before their first scan and therefore before they know they are having twins, so they may be told that their result is 'too high' and suffer all the anxiety that this entails. However, once the scan confirms twins, you can usually be reassured.

Double test and Triple test

These are two very popular blood tests, also known as the Bart's test and Leeds test. You may know about them because they are widely offered to woman expecting single-tons. Unfortunately they are not helpful with multiples. Work is now being carried out to see whether the tests can be applied to twins and higher multiples (for instance by applying a mathematical correction factor to the result), but it will probably be some time before these tests can be considered reliable in these cases.

· *Invasive Tests* ·

The two invasive tests are amniocentesis and CVS.

Amniocentesis

This refers to taking a sample of the amniotic fluid around each baby. It also collects a few of the cells floating free in the fluid and therefore gives information about chromosome abnormalities, such as Down's syndrome, which are commoner in older mothers. You may be offered the test if you are over 38 or 40 years old, or have had a non-invasive test which suggests amniocentesis is a good idea.

Amniocentesis is done in the second three months of pregnancy, usually at about sixteen weeks or more. (Technically, it can be done earlier, but this sometimes makes it more risky.) Because cells have to be grown in the laboratory to yield a result, you may have to wait till nearly twenty weeks before you know the outcome of the test.

The test is done through the abdomen (using local anaesthetic), with a fine needle for each baby, and under ultrasound control to avoid damaging the fetuses or their placentas. To make sure that fluid from both babies is sampled, dye can be injected into one of the amniotic cavities during the test.

The risk of miscarriage from amniocentesis is around 1 per cent. The percentage may be lower if the procedure is carried out using only one needle which goes through the fetal membranes to sample both sacs. Whether one or two needles are used, it is technically difficult to do with twins and higher multiples, so you usually need to be referred to a specialist fetal medicine centre.

Chorionic villus sampling (CVS)

Like amniocentesis, CVS gives information about a baby's chromosomes, but this test samples cells directly from the chorionic villi, which are fragments of the placenta.

CVS is done with a needle through the abdomen or sometimes via the cervix; with multiples it may be done through both. Again, a little local anaesthetic is used and ultrasound control is essential.

The big plus of CVS is that it gives results sooner than amniocentesis, first, because it is done at around eleven to thirteen weeks and, second, because cells don't have to be grown in the lab before being examined. On the minus side, dye cannot be injected during the CVS test. So if the tests yield two lots of genetically identical tissue, it may be impossible to know whether material from both babies has been sampled.

The risk of miscarriage from the CVS is also around 1 per cent. There may be an additional risk of causing abnormalities of the fingers or toes if the test is done before ten weeks. For this reason, it is usually deferred until eleven weeks at the earliest. CVS demands skill and experience in any pregnancy, but especially when carried out with multiples, which is why you will need to be referred to a specialist fetal medicine centre.

· Caring for Yourself during · Pregnancy

Because having multiples puts extra demands on your body and may cause more minor aches and symptoms in pregnancy, it is worth taking good care of yourself – and thereby of your babies too.

Resting

Getting enough rest is an important part of pregnancy. Besides, you are going to be very busy for the next few years. Many pregnant women feel energetic, and others less so. There are no hard and fast rules here, because multiple pregnancies tend to vary far more than do singleton pregnancies. Some women carrying twins have been known to continue with athletic feats, while a few are scarcely able to drag themselves around the shops.

As a rule:

- pelvic floor exercises are essential
- swimming is almost always useful – even if you cannot swim, you will feel nicely buoyant in the water
- you can usually go on doing your usual activities except for such things as contact sports and scuba diving – check with your midwife or doctor if in doubt.

Whatever you do, be sure to pace yourself and listen to your body. It is sometimes said that if your babies kick mainly at night, you are not getting enough rest in the day. There is some logic in this adage since womb space is restricted and there is obviously less room for kicking about when your own muscles are in action all the time.

Going into hospital for a rest

The more babies you are carrying, the more likely you are to have to go into hospital before the due date. The National Study of Triplets and Higher Order Births showed that 95 per cent of women expecting triplets (and all those with quads) were admitted to hospital at least once during their pregnancy.

It was once thought that rest, especially in bed, was in itself beneficial in pregnancy and even that this explained why twins born to privileged middle-class women in Aberdeen were more likely to survive than those of working-class women. We now know this is not the reason. However, rest in hospital is still helpful for some complications and of course also puts you and your babies where the neonatal facilities are.

On the other hand, bed rest has not been shown to reduce the risk of premature labour; nor does it live up to all the claims made for it in the past. Languishing in bed also has its hazards:

- an increased risk of thrombosis in the deep veins of the legs or the pelvis (this is a known complication of pregnancy, especially multiple pregnancy)
- muscle atrophy due to disuse
- a potentially increased risk of osteoporosis (brittle bones), because calcium is lost from the skeleton faster in bed rest.

Osteoporosis causes severe pain in the back or hips. It is unusual in pregnancy but it can happen.

Fortunately, nowadays bed rest is prescribed not so much for its own sake but to enable various complications to be treated or anticipated, for instance by a short period of monitoring in hospital.

Some women are relieved to be in hospital, with its high-tech facilities, and to be away from the demands of a busy home or workplace. But being away from home has obvious drawbacks for you and your family. There are the strange surroundings, the noise, sleep deprivation, the lack of privacy – and hospital food. The latter is often the subject of jokes, but is no laughing matter. In many cases hospital fare is barely adequate for women expecting singletons, let alone those with multiples.

You are more likely to go into hospital happily if there is a good reason, so ask your doctor rather than accepting a stay there unquestioningly. If you live nearby, you may find that you and your obstetrician can reach a compromise which enables you to rest at home. This could really mean rest, with someone else looking after the home and any younger children.

> When my wife went into hospital at 33 weeks for pre-eclampsia, a friend had Amy, then aged two, for most of the day. My boss agreed that I could leave work early to look after her from about 4 p.m. I never thought we'd cope, but we did superbly even if I say so myself. And it was worth it because the twins were born at 35 weeks and all was well.

Healthy eating

The general recommendations for pregnant women are covered in many other books and leaflets, so this section focuses mainly on the special needs of those expecting twins or more.

Your aim is a balanced diet that is enough to nourish you and your babies. However overweight you are to begin with, don't try to lose any weight during your pregnancy. Dieting must wait. Weight gained from eating well-balanced meals is believed to be easier to shed later, if necessary.

During this pregnancy, you can assume that you need 50 per cent to 100 per cent more of important nutrients like iron, calcium, folic acid and vitamin B_{12}. An important exception is vitamin A, which could be harmful to the fetus if taken in excess. (This is the main reason why pregnant women should avoid eating liver or taking cod-liver oil.)

If you eat well and have no complications or other medical conditions, you are unlikely to need vitamin tablets, but this is a controversial area. Some nutritionists believe that the usual recommended daily allowances may be enough to stave off the typical deficiency diseases, like scurvy or pellagra, yet be insufficient for optimum health. If you want to take vitamins while pregnant, check with your midwife, doctor or pharmacist (tell them that you are pregnant). Avoid taking any extra vitamin A in tablet form.

Achieving a balanced diet means eating several portions a day from each of these groups of food:

- *Cereals, breads, rice and pasta* – for carbohydrates (energy), fibre, protein and vitamins. Choose wholemeal and wholegrain products if possible, and avoid too many refined carbohydrates (cakes, biscuits, etc.).

- *Fruit, vegetables and salads* – for vitamins (especially folate (folic acid) and vitamin C), fibre and minerals. Make sure all salads are washed well – there is a risk of toxoplasmosis from soil – and cook vegetables lightly to preserve vitamins.

- *Fish, meat, poultry, eggs, pulses and nuts* – for protein, iron, and vitamin B_{12}. Avoid undercooked meat (because of the risk of toxoplasmosis) and undercooked poultry (because of the risk of salmonella and campylobacter). Eggs should be cooked until the yolk goes hard (to guard against salmonella). If you are a vegetarian, eat plenty of pulses and nuts and use yeast extracts which are rich in B_{12}.

- *Milk, cheese and other dairy products* – for calcium and protein. On average, a woman pregnant with twins or more needs five daily servings to ensure she gets enough calcium. One serving is a yoghurt, a glass of milk, or about 30 grams (1 oz) of cheese. Low-fat milks contain as much calcium as full-fat. Pilchards, sardines and tinned salmon (with the small bones) are also rich in calcium.

All women who are planning to conceive, or are in the first twelve weeks of pregnancy should take a daily folic acid supplement of 400 microgrammes (0.4 mg) to lower the risk of spina bifida and other NTDs. You also need to eat foods rich in folate, like leafy green vegetables, black-eyed peas and folate-enriched bread.

Pregnant women are more at risk from the listeria bacterium and should avoid soft ripened cheeses (like Brie), blue-veined cheeses, pâté of all kinds and cook-chilled foods (unless these are properly heated through).

· *Coping with Common Symptoms* ·

Indigestion and nausea

'Morning' sickness and indigestion or heartburn tend to be worse during a multiple pregnancy, especially when the babies are growing well. These symptoms are thought to be caused by the enlarging bump as well as by hormones, one of which relaxes the muscle at the entrance to the stomach, allowing stomach acid to flow back up the gullet and cause the searing sensation of heartburn.

You can minimize both heartburn and nausea by:

• avoiding fatty or spicy foods, or anything which you know from experience can upset your stomach
• eating frequent small snacks of carbohydrate – dry biscuits, toast, etc.
• drinking milk or taking mild antacids – ask your midwife or chemist (mention that you are pregnant); if you need

anything on prescription, remember that you are exempt from NHS prescription charges during pregnancy

- avoiding heavy meals just before bedtime
- sleeping with two or more pillows, so that your head is higher than your stomach
- avoiding tight clothes – be honest when your jeans no longer fit! When you are pregnant with twins, you may eventually find you even get too large for some maternity clothes.

If you are unable to keep food down, tell your doctor. Some anti-sickness tablets can help in pregnancy, but it is best to check first.

Constipation

The hormone progesterone tends to relax the gut and make bowel action sluggish. You can help avoid constipation by:

- eating plenty of fibre-rich foods
- taking regular exercise, even if it is only a daily walk.

Don't take laxatives unless your doctor or midwife approves. They can be harmful in pregnancy.

Piles (haemorrhoids)

Increased pressure inside the abdomen in the latter half of pregnancy makes piles more common then, especially with twins, but constipation at any time can also bring them on.

Typical symptoms are itching and a painful swelling near the back passage (anus). If you have any bleeding, see your doctor; it may or may not be piles.

- Watch your diet to keep your bowels regular.
- Try not to strain or sit on the toilet for long periods of time.

- When you need to go, go then. Don't put it off till later.
- Use soft toilet paper. If you already have itching or a lump, wash often. Wet wipes kept in your handbag are useful when out and about.
- Check with your doctor or chemist before using any of the available over-the-counter remedies for haemorrhoids.

Backache

Low back pain is common in twin pregnancy, first, because the extra load puts the spine under greater mechanical strain and, second, because the abdominal muscles are more fully stretched and cannot do their bit to stabilize the spine. In addition, the hormone relaxin, which softens the ligaments in the spine and elsewhere (and is therefore useful during labour and childbirth), can make minor aches and injuries more likely during pregnancy.

- Try to keep your spine straight. Avoid standing with the small of the back fully curved in the typical pregnant posture. Instead, tuck your buttocks in and tilt the front of your pelvis up.
- Wearing flattish shoes is better for your posture.
- Don't bend your back when bending forwards. (In any case, you will eventually be unable to.) Bend at the knees instead when picking anything off the floor.
- Take care when getting into and out of bed, especially in late pregnancy. Roll on to your side first then put your feet on the floor before sitting up.
- Avoid press-ups, sit-ups and heavy lifting. Don't rearrange furniture unaided and carry your toddler only when absolutely necessary.
- Go swimming – it is one of the things you can often enjoy until late in pregnancy, if you can find a large enough

swimsuit. Some women who are pregnant with twins find they outgrow many maternity swimsuits.

• Specific back exercises can both prevent and relieve backache, for instance getting on all fours and alternately arching your back and letting it sag. Your antenatal teacher can tell you about others.

• When your back hurts, a warm bath (not hot), a gentle massage from your partner and the odd paracetamol can all help. Avoid other drugs unless you've checked with your doctor.

Varicose veins

Because of your growing bump and your hormonal changes, prominent or bulging leg veins, with or without aching, are common in pregnancy. You won't necessarily get varicose veins; family history is a factor too.

• When sitting, keep your feet up on a stool or coffee table rather than dangling down.

• Don't stand for long periods of time. If you must, keep moving your legs.

• Walking is a good form of exercise and will keep blood flowing rather than stagnating in your leg veins.

• Maternity support tights help.

Insomnia

During the last few weeks of pregnancy, as your bump becomes increasingly large and thoughts go whizzing round your head, sleeplessness can be a real nuisance.

• Wind down to bedtime with a restful routine. Avoid coffee, tea and caffeinated soft drinks in the evening.

- Make yourself as comfortable as you can. Lying on your side with the help of a pillow or two to support your abdomen may be the best position (however, you can get fed up with it).

- Use the relaxation technique you learned in antenatal classes.

- If you are worried about something, bring the issue out into the open and discuss it with your partner, or jot down the questions you'd like to ask your midwife when you next see her.

Skin changes

Stretch marks are common after a twin pregnancy but they are not inevitable and many women don't get them. However, in the last month or two, itchy skin on the lower abdomen or the back bothers many pregnant women. This is thought to be caused by dryness and stretching of the skin.

- Avoid scratching if possible, because it releases the chemical histamine into the skin, which makes itching worse.

- Keep your skin smooth with bath oils and body lotions, preferably unperfumed. The worst areas may respond to Vaseline or calamine lotion.

- Baths should be warm rather than hot.

- If you get itching all over the body or in unusual places (for instance, on your hands and feet), contact your doctor, especially if you also have dark urine or pale stools. You may have cholestasis of pregnancy, a rare condition that is no more common in twin pregnancy. It needs to be recognized promptly, however, as it has the potential to cause stillbirth. The usual treatment is close monitoring of the mother combined with an earlier delivery of the babies.

Swollen hands and feet

Mild swelling of the feet, and to some extent the fingers, is not unusual, especially on a hot day in the later stages of pregnancy. However, you should always bring it to the notice of your midwife or doctor just in case it is a sign of pre-eclampsia.

As long as all's well, just try to make things easier and

● wear comfortable shoes
● rest with your feet up when possible
● avoid standing unnecessarily
● wear maternity support tights
● remove rings before your fingers get too podgy.

Sex

There can be problems with sex during pregnancy for several reasons. You may be tired or uncomfortable, or perhaps you've just gone off the idea, especially if you are having a lot of physical symptoms or find it difficult to adapt to your impending role as a mother (as tends to be the case in a first pregnancy). Alternatively, your partner may have gone off it: while some men find the pregnant shape appealing, others do not. Perhaps you or your partner is afraid of hurting the babies; you may have noticed that they often kick a lot more after intercourse.

If you do feel like it, there is no reason why you should not have intercourse during your multiple pregnancy, provided you have no complications, such as premature contractions or vaginal bleeding, and have not been told by your doctor to abstain. Obstetricians vary a bit as to what they consider safe in multiple pregnancies. If in doubt, check.

That said, your most taxing problem could be one of logistics. As the weeks go by, you will have to use your

imagination to get close to each other. You may find you
prefer to give up on penetrative sex and use other means of
giving and receiving pleasure.

· *Preparing Yourself for Twins* ·
or More

As you approach the big day, emotional preparation can be
as important as taking physical care of yourself. By now, you
and your nearest and dearest may feel well adjusted to the
idea of having more than one baby, but, unless there are
twins in your family or immediate circle of friends, you cannot appreciate all the implications.

As several nurses and midwives have found out, you don't
know what it is like to have multiple babies until you experience it at first hand. Research by midwifery advisor Jane
Spillman for TAMBA underlines this point. Around a fifth of
the mothers in one of her studies were health professionals
themselves, yet it was only when they themselves were
expecting multiples that they realized they didn't have all the
answers and needed far more information and advice.

There is a lot you can do in the time you have left, which is
one of the many advantages of diagnosing multiples early in
pregnancy rather than in the delivery suite.

1   Attend antenatal and parentcraft classes in good time.
    Multiples tend to arrive early and often with little warn-
    ing. Even if yours stay the course, you may not feel up to
    travelling to and from the hospital in the last few weeks.
    If you try to complete antenatal classes at least a month
    ahead of women expecting singletons, you probably won't
    miss much.

    Few hospitals have antenatal courses aimed at
    women expecting multiples (though when they do, they

are much appreciated) so you may find the content of the classes geared exclusively towards single births. This is something Jane Spillman's work confirms, and it makes it very hard for expectant mothers to get appropriate information. In antenatal classes, you can always speak up and ask whether particular aspects mentioned will apply to you.

Make sure that you visit the special care baby unit (SCBU) on your tour of the hospital, as your babies have a higher chance of having to spend some time there. Find out too about what your hospital offers in the way of pain relief (in the next chapter there is more on this and other aspects of labour, including caesareans).

If you live within striking distance of London, you may be interested in attending one or more of the MBF's prenatal evening meetings for prospective parents (and grandparents) of multiples; contact the MBF direct.

2   Meet others in your area who already have twins or who are expecting them. Contact TAMBA direct if the hospital cannot put you in touch with your local group.

Twins' clubs can help you make friends and find out more about the practicalities of caring for twins and you will also get the chance to borrow books and perhaps to see a video of a twin birth if you and your partner would like to. The clubs are often also excellent sources of good second-hand baby equipment.

3   Try to prepare your family for the big event. Seeing the scan (or a photo of it) and attending clinic appointments can help bring the reality home to your partner, but it can also create worries which need to be talked through so that together you can develop a coping strategy.

Some men aren't good at expressing their emotions, but your partner may be just as concerned as you are about the health of your babies. He may have his own anxieties too. As a father of twins, his role is likely to be more hands-on than it is for most fathers of singletons. How will he cope with his job as well as lend you practical help? Can he take leave from work? Will he now have to work harder to make up for the loss of your income?

If the pregnancy was unplanned, how will you both embrace your new status as parents – not just of one baby, but of two or more? It can be double the shock if you hadn't intended to conceive yet (or at all). As well as discussing matters together, you may both benefit from talking things over with someone outside the family: a GP, midwife, psychologist (ask your GP) or a stress counsellor at work.

Grandparents may need educating to understand what you are going through. The older generation can be unduly pessimistic about twins because the outlook was bleak in their day. On the other hand, grandparents sometimes have unrealistic notions about how wonderful twins, triplets or more can be. They will no doubt be proud and want to brag, but they also need to appreciate that you will need help, preferably without too much meddling or telling you how to do things all the time. A fortunate few may find a grandparent is able to help with the cost of an *au pair*, maternity nurse or mother's help.

The birth of two or more siblings at once is bound to be a difficult time for any children you already have and can alter their lives fundamentally. Give your older child as much time and attention as you can now and work out ahead of time what you will do when you go into hospital. You will find lots more ideas on relationships in chapter 8.

4   Make plans for your own job if you have one. Will you return to work after the birth? You cannot know now

exactly how you will feel – even if you're fairly sure you are leaving for good, it is sometimes best from your point of view to tell your employer that you are undecided. Once a permanent replacement is ensconced in your office, it could be impossible to return.

Perhaps you are now contemplating a change, to a part-time job or one that fits in better with a double dose of parenting. This may be a good time, before you have your babies in tow, to explore a few possibilities that involve new training.

Your employer must give you time off work to attend for antenatal care, which generally means antenatal classes too. However, whatever you can do to minimize the impact on your work could be appreciated. Can you make up the work some other time?

If this is your first pregnancy, you may want to press on with work until you drop (or your twins do). Many women prefer to take their paid maternity leave after the birth rather than before, but this is unrealistic with a multiple pregnancy. Most experts suggest that you stop working a bit sooner if you are expecting twins or more. Other things being equal, it is reasonable to go on maternity leave from the twenty-ninth week of pregnancy until the babies are six months old – at least. You can find out about your entitlements to statutory maternity pay, maternity allowance, child benefit and one-parent benefit from the booklet 'Babies and Benefits', available at post offices, antenatal clinics and from the DSS.

Much depends on how your pregnancy is progressing – multiple pregnancies vary a lot – and of course on your particular job. The Health and Safety at Work (Amendment) Regulations 1994 require employers to take account of particular risks to pregnant employees and new mothers. If risks cannot be avoided by other means, working hours or conditions have to change. Or, if this proves impossible, you must be given paid leave for as long as necessary to protect your health and that of your babies. You can get more information from the Health and Safety Executive.

Whatever your job, severe morning sickness may lead you to negotiate a later start to your working day. Even if you have a sedentary job, you may get very tired. A lunchtime or early afternoon rest, taken lying down, can help counteract fatigue and may also improve placental blood flow. Don't be shy about asking for this: you have a role in looking after the next generation. Besides, employers are now obliged to provide rest facilities for pregnant (or breast-feeding) workers.

The journey to and from work can become difficult. As many heavily pregnant women discover, you can practically give birth on a crowded commuter train before anyone bats an eyelid, let alone gives up their seat. The problem may be solved if you are allowed a parking space, so that you can drive to work – as long as the seat-belt still fits over your bump, which it may not do for much longer.

5   You may like to start stroking, talking or singing to your babies. It is now known that babies can feel, hear, and even see long before birth. In the last few months of pregnancy, fetuses see well enough to distinguish light from dark. They certainly respond to being prodded at five months and may react to touch from as early as eight weeks or so, at which time each baby is barely two centimetres long. Research also suggests that in the last few months of pregnancy babies respond to sound, moving their bodies gently in time to the rhythm of their mother's voice.

It is not known whether shaping a baby's prenatal environment affects later development, but it may. A few experts, such as Elizabeth Noble (Director of Women's Health Resources, Cape Cod, Massachusetts), advocate talking to your babies in the womb and explaining to them that they must learn to share and to be kind to each other. While this is not proven to make any difference, if you feel so inclined it may help you to bond with your babies. You and your partner may also find it fun.

It has been suggested that women under serious emotional stress tend to have hyperactive babies, though this has not been convincingly shown to have a cause-and-effect relationship. Besides, you cannot become placid just because you want to be, though you can certainly try to unwind with relaxation techniques.

6   Read the next few chapters and think ahead about practical matters. Will you want to breast-feed? How will you manage in the first few days at home? Where will the babies sleep? Get a minimum of baby equipment organized. Many mothers-to-be are superstitious, and there could also be financial reasons not to stock up on everything in advance, but you will need some items from the earliest days. You may be able to borrow enough from friends.

7   Start thinking of names and draw up a short (or long?) list of your favourites for both boys and girls, unless you already know from a scan which you are expecting. This may save you from making hasty decisions after the birth, or calling your babies 'Pink Blanket' and 'White Blanket', for three days until you and your partner agree.

A child's name is an integral part of his individuality and personality and choosing names for multiples, while double or treble the fun, needs care. Names like Kirsten and Christine which sound very similar will prove difficult at school. Try also to avoid two or more names with the same initial (Thomas and Theresa), and rhyming names (Jenny and Penny). Thinking of how the names might sound when abbreviated will help you steer clear of Amy and Jamie, for instance.

Matching names (Jade and Pearl, Holly and Ivy) might seem witty at the time but could be deeply resented later. Names which are very different in length (like Christopher and Ben) are often a good idea but sometimes pose problems at a stage when the children are learning to write.

Consider too what the names sound like together. When talking about your children to someone who doesn't know them, Lily and Mary may be mistaken for the single name Lilian Mary. (Reversing the order will not help, because Mary and Lily sounds like Marian Lily.)

You may like to name your twins or triplets in reverse alphabetical order, so that the first-born is called Natasha and the second-born Andrew. Then at least Andrew will come first in something, which could count for a lot in later childhood.

One or two families have gone even further, using different surnames, one from the mother and the other from the father. This could work if the mother uses her maiden name anyway.

8 Take old wives' tales with a pinch of salt, whether they are about childbirth in general or multiples in particular. You may have heard that labour is the most painful experience on earth, or that the girl of a boy–girl pair of twins is always sterile. Neither is true. Discount these and other myths that can destroy your peace of mind.

9 You are bound to have a few questions, worries or doubts, but the more unresolved problems you have, the less you will enjoy your pregnancy. Although clinics and surgeries are busy places, you should consult your doctor or midwife if you have medical queries. Medics tend to shy away from patients with long written lists (said to be a sure sign of a hypochondriac!), so be assertive if necessary. Also, prioritize. Don't leave your most burning question till last; the doctor may have been called away by then.

Unfortunately, those caring for you may be unable to answer all your questions because they have little experience of multiples. In these cases, check the contents of this book or ask TAMBA. If any of the professionals you meet need more information, you can also put them in touch with TAMBA or MBF, each of which has a role to play in educating the professionals.

10 Could anything more be done? There is mounting evidence that social and psychological support antenatally can help avert postnatal depression. It is the quality of care rather than the sheer quantity of antenatal appointments that matter. If you feel you are not getting the emotional attention you need, make it known. If you are a family in difficulties, or anticipate particular problems in caring for your babies, early social work involvement could make all the difference. It is best not to be too proud.

For some women, on the other hand, it is just a question of time. Maybe you won't entirely adjust until after the event. A few mothers resent twins, and grieve for the cosy one-to-one relationship they might have had with a single baby. Once they get over this, great joys are in store.

I only had six weeks at home with my first son, so I was going to take much longer off work after my second baby and really get to know him or her. I was also determined to breast-feed for longer. But my plans were completely shot by the fact that the second baby was not one but two. I now think they are the best thing that ever happened to me. But it was many months before I got used to the idea of them being twins.

Chapter Three

THE BIG DAY: LABOUR AND BIRTH

Unless your hospital makes special antenatal provision for women expecting more than one baby, some of what you are told about labour and birth in antenatal classes will not apply to you, and you will be left wondering just what it will be like when you give birth. There are several reassuring facts you should know at the outset:

- Labour with twins is not twice as painful or twice as long as with singletons. In fact, it can even be less uncomfortable because the babies tend to be a bit smaller.
- No matter how many babies you are having, the cervix needs to dilate fully only once, so you go through just one first stage of labour.
- Although the birth is more hazardous for twins (especially for the second baby), with proper care it can be made safer.

It is very natural to be concerned about labour, how it will be for your babies and for yourself. While you should not underestimate the potential difficulties, it is an advantage not to be fearful. This is where being well informed helps. If anything is worrying you, ask your doctor or midwife early on. The answer may make you feel a lot easier in your mind.

In general, the more relaxed you are, the better your experience of birth can be. This is probably because emotions such as fear and anxiety are intimately linked with circulating hormones like adrenalin, which makes muscles tense up.

Some midwives even claim that a tense jaw during labour mirrors an unyielding perineum. You may well find that on the day you will be much happier and calmer than you anticipated. Women tend to rise to the occasion of birth. Hormones again, perhaps?

· *Premature Labour* ·

You need to know about premature labour and how to recognize it because twins and higher multiples have a disconcerting tendency to arrive early. In the first three months of pregnancy, vital organs are formed, while during the next six months they grow at a phenomenal rate. If you consider this then you will realize just how important prematurity can be.

Normally 'full term' for twins is 37 weeks, while triplets often arrive at 34 weeks and quads at 33 weeks, as mentioned in the last chapter. Anything earlier than this is considered premature, but obviously there are differences of degree. Twins born a few days short of 37 weeks don't face the same dangers as those born at 28 weeks.

- About 30 per cent of twins are pre-term, while the figure for singletons is only 10 per cent.
- About 30 per cent of triplets are born before 32 weeks and 10 per cent are born before 28 weeks.
- For quads, there is less information available, but nearly half deliver before 32 weeks, and 25 per cent before 28 weeks.

Which babies arrive early?

Premature labour is more common in identical (MZ) twins, especially if there is only one chorionic membrane and if they are boys. The reason is not clear, but funnily enough male singletons are also more likely to deliver early.

If you are expecting twins in your first pregnancy, you are more likely to go into labour prematurely than if this is your second or subsequent pregnancy. It is sometimes said that in premature labour the membranes rupture early with identical twins, but contractions start first with non-identicals.

What causes prematurity?

During a multiple pregnancy, there are on average more contractions, mostly of the Braxton-Hicks type. These are low-strength contractions which are often described as the womb 'getting into training'. It is not surprising that in multiple pregnancy the muscle of the uterus is a bit more taut and irritable, as it were – after all, it has more to contend with.

In themselves, Braxton-Hicks contractions don't spell premature labour, but they can herald it. Premature labour involves not just uterine contractions, but the cervix changing and beginning to dilate.

Nobody really knows what starts premature labour – or any labour, come to that. It is not simply a question of the womb being stretched to capacity. If it were, more twins would be born at about 28 to 30 weeks, when the size of the uterus approaches that of a singleton at term. Nor does mere bulk explain the well-known link between premature labour and slow growth in the womb.

There are various theories. Perhaps with multiples the fetal membranes (the chorion and amnion) simply produce more prostaglandins, natural chemicals which are known to stimulate the womb muscles to contract. Or maybe the uterus is more sensitive to other hormones, like oxytocin which is released by the pituitary gland and causes strong uterine contractions (a synthetic version is sometimes given by injection during labour to speed it up). Sometimes labour is triggered by complications such as hydramnios, or by infection. Research is being done into the possible role of mild infections in late pregnancy, which could perhaps cause labour by releasing enzymes into the chorion and amnion.

Symptoms of premature labour

Whatever actually starts things off, it is vital to be aware of the possible symptoms. These are basically the same as those of any labour, so you may start getting:

- regular contractions (every ten to fifteen minutes)
- pain in the pelvis or back
- an unusually heavy feeling in the pelvis
- blood or mucus from the vagina (either of which can indicate changes in the cervix)
- clear fluid from the vagina (this usually indicates ruptured membranes).

If you have any of these symptoms, contact the labour ward. If you are not sure of the significance of your symptoms, check with the labour ward anyway. In your situation, it is wise to ignore reassuring noises from friends who have singletons. It is far better to raise a false alarm, especially with multiples, than to leave things too late. If you need any further incentive to act fast, remember that labour could be over very quickly, especially if your babies are small, and your babies may be more vulnerable than singletons.

Dealing with premature labour

As long as the babies are growing well, the uterus is the best incubator available. So what can be done when premature labour threatens?

If you suspect premature labour, one thing you should do is avoid sex (and any strenuous activity), at least until you have checked with your doctor. Intercourse puts pressure on the cervix and the prostaglandins in semen may be enough to tip the balance and trigger full-blown labour.

Over the years, many measures have been devised to prevent or halt premature labour, but they haven't proved to be reliable with twins and higher-order pregnancies.

- Bed rest takes the weight off the cervix and helps improve placental blood flow, but on the whole hospital bed rest is of doubtful benefit.

- Cervical suture (encircling the cervix with a strong stitch) has not been shown to be beneficial either except in special circumstances where the cervix is lax.

- Drugs like salbutamol and the other so-called sympathomimetics (ritodrine, feneterol, terbutaline) have been used, either by mouth or by injection. So have alcohol, nifedipine, magnesium sulphate and indomethacin (an anti-inflammatory drug), but there is little evidence that any of these are helpful in multiple pregnancy.

However, the research results are a little conflicting. Some French specialists claim success in preventing twins from arriving very early (before 28 to 30 weeks) with a belt-and-braces approach, using both rest and sympathomimetics to prevent premature labour, but this is unlikely to help the vast majority of women expecting twins.

In fact the overall proportion of babies born too soon has hardly changed in the last two or three decades, but premature babies – multiples and singletons – are doing a lot better because of other medical advances. For instance, it is now possible to give babies steroids before birth to speed up the maturation of their lungs.

So what is the point of doing anything about premature labour? Maybe the best argument in favour of going to hospital early with suspected premature labour is that it enables your babies to get swift specialized care, before, during and after birth.

· *Labour* ·

Whether your babies arrive on time or early, your labour is likely to be more high-tech than with singletons, so that complications can be spotted and treated promptly. Some women may find this medicalization of childbirth off-putting, or even plain disappointing. Surely pregnancy and birth are natural, so why treat the process like the advanced stage of a dangerous disease?

Over the last ten to fifteen years, women have been able to reclaim the experience of becoming mothers and have had greater choice in childbirth. Women and their midwives have become more vocal and there has been something of a backlash against the traditional mechanistic – and often paternalistic – pattern of obstetric care. Midwives are once again the professionals with the lead role in normal pregnancy and labour. Meanwhile, doctors are increasingly questioning the part they themselves play and the results of their actions.

During this time, medical intervention in labour has become less intrusive. Some of the changes are very tangible. For instance, induction of labour at term is now much less usual, the use of stirrups is rare and many more women are free to walk around in labour than they were twenty years ago.

The snag is that the human species is really only geared to producing one offspring at a time. Twin and higher-order pregnancies are not normal. This has to be accepted by mothers – and by midwives, a few of whom are still keen to exclude obstetricians until the last possible moment in labour.

Good teamwork is the best approach for a woman in labour with twins. It may be that your twins will be delivered by a midwife, but with an obstetrician in attendance too. Labour is more traumatic for multiples, particularly when they are small or premature, and some are both. There is also a higher risk of cord prolapse and abnormal presentation, for instance, and on rare occasions twins can even lock: their presenting parts wedge together and make normal delivery impossible. For all these reasons, you are about twice as likely to need help in labour, either with forceps or a caesarean, than with a singleton birth.

That is not to say the birth won't be a joyous event, just that you should be prepared for it to be different from having one baby. And if your doctor proposes any intervention in labour, you are of course entitled to ask why.

Who will be at the birth?

Multiple births can pull a big crowd. Apart from the midwife and obstetrician, there will often be an anaesthetist for you and a paediatrician for each baby. There could also be many other nurses, midwives, junior doctors and possibly medical students, all determined not to miss the event. One mother counted 22 people in the labour room at one point during her recent twin birth!

Large numbers can be very off-putting and some women may feel that their big moment has turned into some kind of show. Multiple births are of course unusual and health professionals in training need to learn about them, but if you find the audience disturbing, say so. Tell your doctor or midwife, preferably as early on as possible. Some of the observers may also be embarrassed and will leave quite happily once asked.

You can decide about this, and other preferences you may have, in advance with your partner or birth companion. In the overwhelming excitement of labour, it helps to have someone to speak up for you.

Method of delivery

Caesareans are more common with twins. (The word comes from the Latin *caesus*, from the verb *caedere*, to cut, though commonly believed to refer to Julius Caesar – but his mother didn't have a caesarean!) In the UK, about 28 per cent of twins are delivered this way, compared with 10 per cent of singletons.

Triplets and higher multiples

Higher multiples are even likelier to be born by caesarean. The more babies you are carrying, the likelier it is that you will need intervention. Quads and more are almost always born by caesarean.

What is considered the best method varies with locality. In the USA, 90 per cent of triplets arrive by caesarean, but only 14 per cent in South Africa. Within the UK there is a little variation from one hospital to another, but, over all, most triplets are born by caesarean. It may be reasonable to aim for a vaginal delivery if the first baby is head-down, but the trouble is that the way the second and third babies are lying can change during labour; they may therefore need help in a hurry. Under the circumstances, there is logic in having them all by caesarean.

Presentation of twins

How your twins lie in the womb towards the end of your pregnancy is a major factor in deciding the most appropriate method of delivery. In about three-quarters of twin pregnancies, the first twin is head-down, in what is known as a vertex or cephalic presentation.

About 40 per cent of twins are both head-down. Almost all of these may deliver normally, though their heart rates will be closely monitored in labour for any signs of distress. If you had a caesarean for a previous birth, there is still a chance that your twins can be born vaginally, just as long as your last caesarean was for a one-off reason, not for a permanent condition (for instance, a small pelvis).

In about 33 per cent of twins, the first is head-down but the second is breech (bottom-down), which is where things start getting complicated. The danger for a breech baby is that he cannot breathe as soon, because his head is born last. A breech baby is sometimes turned around in labour, a procedure called 'internal version'. If your second twin is breech, you may still be able to have a vaginal delivery, unless:

- you had a previous caesarean, for whatever reason (it may not be safe to turn a breech around in a womb that has a caesarean scar)

- you are in the USA, where the rate of medical intervention is higher

- there are complications, like fetal distress.

In about 25 per cent of twins, the first baby is a breech. Here a caesarean is often done without going into labour at all. On the other hand, if all is well you may be allowed to labour for a while to see if there is any progress. It all depends on your individual circumstances and what your obstetrician believes would be best for your babies.

If a caesarean is needed, both babies are born this way. It is unusual – though not unheard of – for the first twin to be born through the vagina and the second to have a caesarean for a problem that crops up in labour.

Forceps are also about twice as common for twin births, either to rotate the baby's head into a better position, or to get him out more quickly if distressed. Sometimes a ventouse (a suction instrument applied to a baby's head) can do this job instead, but it is not used for very small or premature babies because they are too vulnerable.

As you can see, exactly what happens depends not just on how the babies lie, but on factors which vary from woman to woman. An ultrasound may, for instance, have shown placenta praevia, a condition in which one or other placenta lies so low down in the womb that normal labour is impossibly dangerous.

Obstetric practice also varies a little from hospital to hospital, so you need to discuss with your specialist what is likely to happen in your case. Incidentally, the percentages given above are only approximate and they don't add up to 100 because not all babies are breech or vertex. Some are transverse, which means that they lie horizontally across the uterus and therefore require a caesarean for safe delivery.

Pain relief

There are several methods, including:

- 'gas and air' (the gas is nitrous oxide. Entonox is nitrous oxide and oxygen)
- pethidine by injection (if given within two hours or so of delivery, this may affect the babies' breathing just after birth, especially the second twin's)
- pudendal block (local anaesthetic is injected deep into the pelvis; it is sometimes used for forceps delivery, though an epidural is usually preferable)
- epidural injection (described below).

There are also drug-free methods, such as transcutaneous nerve stimulation (TNS or TENS). Relaxation should not be dismissed either – it is helpful in early labour.

Before they go into labour, some women decide that they want as little pain relief as possible, or even none. A few think that only a truly natural (often very painful) birth is the right way to deliver a baby, and that anything less is an inglorious cop-out.

However, pain can be downright counter-productive. It can result in uncoordinated contractions which slow down labour and reduce placental blood flow to your babies. Pain also inhibits your own stomach from emptying, increasing the risk of your bringing up acid. This is dangerous, for instance if you suddenly need a general anaesthetic.

Control of labour pain has many advantages, not least of which is that you may feel calmer and better able to enjoy labour once pain no longer intrudes.

Epidurals

In an epidural, local anaesthetic is injected into the spinal epidural space around the nerve fibres to deaden them during labour. Successful use of the technique demands an excellent anaesthetic service and hospitals differ in how much of this they provide.

There is little doubt that the epidural has been the greatest advance in pain control in the last generation. It is the only method – barring general anaesthetic – that can totally abolish labour pains and it has special advantages for women with multiples:

- An epidural is ideal for a breech delivery.

- The second baby can change position after the first twin is born. Turning him without an epidural or general anaesthetic would be excruciating.

- With an epidural in place any other sort of intervention (via forceps or a caesarean) that may be needed can be done without a potentially dangerous delay.

- A caesarean under epidural rather than general anaesthetic allows you and your partner not to miss the first precious moments with your babies.

As a woman expecting twins, you may therefore be advised, encouraged, cajoled or even told to have an epidural during labour. One or two obstetricians have even been known to refuse to undertake the care of a woman with twins unless she agrees to one. This is a bit extreme, but there are such good reasons for having an epidural for twin deliveries that the motives are understandable. More to the point, perhaps, women who have had epidurals are often very pleased with their effect.

The procedure

You will be lying on your side, with your knees and head bent. The anaesthetist will inject a little local anaesthetic into the skin of your back, which stings momentarily.

Then he or she guides a very fine tube between two vertebrae (lumber vertebrae number 3 and number 4) in the middle of the back and into the epidural space, through which nerves travel outwards from the spinal cord to the rest of the body. These nerves carry sensation back to the spinal cord and up to the brain, where pain is ultimately 'felt'. To check that all is well, a test dose of anaesthetic is used at this stage.

Once in place, an epidural can be topped up with long-acting anaesthetic as needed, tailoring the dose to your requirements. For a caesarean, for instance, a fairly large dose is used, but for a vaginal delivery the anaesthetic can be allowed to wear off a bit so that you can feel the urge to push in time with your contractions. Epidurals can also be used for pain relief after delivery.

The downside

You may have some worries about epidurals, but about 90 per cent of them are satisfactory overall. Recent research shows that back pain, which some women think of as a complication of labour, is not more common after epidural. However, nothing in medicine is without some disadvantage, and epidurals do have potential problems; roughly in descending order of frequency these are:

- Blood pressure tends to fall with an epidural, so you will need a drip in your hand or arm. The drawback is that you will be a bit less mobile during labour as a result.

- The most common difficulty is that the epidural may not work completely, though this is less likely with an experienced anaesthetist. Occasionally, numbness is patchy or only on one side of the body, which means that another method of pain relief has to be considered.

- While an epidural is being set up, there is a small risk of the needle piercing a membrane called the dura. This releases a few drops of cerebro-spinal fluid (CSF). It may sound frightening, but all it means in practice is that you may get a headache for a few days. Although it is not generally serious, the headache is pretty bad, and worse when sitting up. This obviously makes it harder to look after and enjoy your newborn babies, but it passes.

Vaginal delivery

Twin births usually follow three main stages when delivery is through the vagina.

The first stage: dilatation of the cervix

During this time, contractions build up in strength and frequency. A baby's heart rate is one indication of how he is coping with labour. To make sure your babies are not being distressed by the experience, their heart rates will be monitored continuously throughout. Usually the first twin has a scalp electrode attached to his head (it can also be attached to the bottom of a breech baby), while the second twin is monitored externally via a sensor strapped to your abdomen. Thus both heart rates are monitored electronically.

With all this equipment in place, especially if you have an epidural as well, you will not be as mobile in labour as you might have liked. Don't count on wanting to walk around much, however. By the time you get to term, you could be large and uncomfortable and may want to do all the lying down you can.

How long does the first stage take? A first-time mother (known as a primigravida or primip) tends to have a slower labour, but it is impossible to be dogmatic here. In general the labour takes no longer than with a single baby. These days you are not left to languish in established labour; it tends to get speeded up medically if progress is poor.

The second stage: birth of the babies themselves

For the first baby's head to emerge, you will need to push along with the contractions and with your midwife's or doctor's instructions. If you have an epidural which numbs most or all the sensation, watching the monitor can help you synchronize your efforts with the contractions.

In most cases, the rest of the body follows swiftly, and the cord is clamped. If necessary, the second twin's membranes are then ruptured artificially at this point. His birth usually follows within 20 minutes or less, thanks to some more pushing on your part.

Until recently, the interval between first and second twin was rarely allowed to extend beyond 30 minutes for fear that the second baby might go dangerously short of oxygen. This can indeed happen, but nowadays it is clear that a longer interval can be safe, as long as the baby continues to be monitored closely throughout. Naturally, though, you will not want too long a wait!

The third stage: delivery of the placentas

After the second twin is born and his cord is clamped, both placentas are delivered. They are either expelled naturally or delivered by gentle pulling on the cords. Occasionally the first twin's placenta arrives before the second twin is born.

Caesarean section

Since around a quarter of all twins in the UK are delivered by caesarean section, and you might not otherwise be told much about the procedure, it is worth focusing on what could happen.

A caesarean can be carried out as a planned procedure, without your going into labour at all. This is known as an elective caesarean and might be needed because of the way your twins are lying or in the case of placenta praevia, for example. A caesarean can also be done in an emergency, usually because one or other baby has become distressed during labour, but sometimes because of some other problem.

Either way, the technique is much the same. What is more, the order in which your twins are born with a caesarean is the same as if they had been delivered through the vagina, although many women imagine the order might be reversed.

Caesareans are normally done through a horizontal cut about 15 cm (6 inches) long, below or near the bikini line. You will be lying on your back, slightly tilted to one side. The obstetrician carrying out the procedure usually tilts you away from him or herself (the assistant will be the one to get wet feet from your copious amounts of amniotic fluid). You will need a catheter for a few hours, possibly till the next day, to drain urine from your bladder. Most women don't find this uncomfortable.

The operation itself will not start till you are properly anaesthetized, either with a general anaesthetic or with an epidural which has taken full effect. If you have an epidural, your partner can normally remain with you throughout the caesarean, though he will be asked to stay near your head, where he can sit and talk to you without getting in the doctors' way.

With an epidural you don't usually feel a thing apart from a gentle rummaging sensation, or perhaps a little pulling, once the surgeon has got through the skin. Generally this is not unpleasant, but if you find it painful, say so. You won't usually see anything either, because a sterile drape is erected as a screen at about the level of your chest, but of course you hear and see your babies as soon as they emerge. As long as they don't need immediate medical help, you can have one or both put on to your chest to let them suckle or just to hold them close. In fact you can usually hold or touch them momentarily even if they need to go to the special care unit.

If you have a general anaesthetic, your partner is not normally allowed to stay with you, but you could ask the staff. He might want to be there, if only to take pictures of your babies' arrival. Alternatively, he may be allowed in as soon as they are born, to see them and hold them before you wake up.

For technical reasons, or through shortage of experienced anaesthetists, a few women who have an epidural may still end up having a general anaesthetic for their caesarean. This is understandably a disappointment, especially if it has been promised that an epidural will take care of every eventuality.

You'll stay in hospital a bit longer after a caesarean, perhaps up to a week or so. And you are not exempt from postnatal exercises. Since your pelvic muscles have to work hard in the last few weeks of pregnancy, you still have to get them in shape after the birth.

The downside

Caesareans often get a bad press. The modern caesarean is very safe but it has its drawbacks:

- you feel more tired after the birth
- you usually lose blood from the vagina for longer afterwards

- it is harder to look after babies, and to breast-feed them, when you are recovering from surgery yourself.

> The next day I felt really faint when I went to the loo. I was told I'd lost a litre of blood during the caesarean. All the other mothers on the ward were able to push the cots on wheels about, but I couldn't for about 48 hours and even then I had trouble managing two. Not all the nurses understood the difficulties of coping with two babies after a caesarean.

You cannot expect to feel as well as you would if your abdomen hadn't been cut and tiredness is perhaps the biggest disadvantage. This can really matter when you have to cope with multiples and need all the strength and energy you can summon. Research done by TAMBA's midwifery advisor Jane Spillman suggests that women who have had caesareans for twins and more feel less well in themselves after the birth and may have a slightly higher risk of post-natal depression. Therefore, a caesarean, like any operation, should clearly not be done without good reason. On the other hand, none of the minuses should deter one from having a caesarean when it is necessary.

Some women feel cheated out of their experience of childbirth, as if it's not a proper delivery unless you push a baby out yourself. Disappointment is perhaps normal if you had set your heart on a natural birth or had not considered the possibility of anything else.

Antenatal classes don't teach much about caesareans, so no wonder many women are unprepared. I believe they would feel more positive if they knew more, however. Insensitive remarks from other mothers on the postnatal ward along the lines of 'Poor you', as if something awful had happened, can be very upsetting; a little more information for them about caesareans might not go amiss either.

In fact, many women are very happy with their caesareans. Research shows that, over all, one woman in twelve expecting her first baby actually wants a caesarean, but the figure goes up to one in five for women who have previously had one. Those in the know agree: female obstetricians often ask for a caesarean for themselves.

Women, like myself, who have their babies under epidural tend to be the most satisfied, often describing their experience in glowing terms and commenting on the supremely happy atmosphere during the birth.

> I hadn't even wanted an epidural, let alone a caesarean, but it was excellent. After the birth I was crying but this was because I was so happy. My husband and two of the staff seemed overwhelmed, too. Yes, the day my sons were born by caesarean was the best day of my life. It was then, and it still is true now, ten years on.

If you have a general anaesthetic, you may feel groggy for a day or so and you will certainly miss the big event and those early moments. On the other hand, it is only a few hours in the life of your children. Finally, you could try crowing over anyone who implies that you didn't have a proper birth. Unlike them, you can now sit down in comfort.

Twin births at home

Don't even consider it. Some doctors quip that women asking for a home birth for twins need to see a psychiatrist, not an obstetrician. Others may simply tell the woman to stop being so selfish.

Seriously, though, given the risks twins face, there are persuasive medical reasons which make home births totally unsuitable.

- The risk of malpresentation, cord prolapse, post-partum haemorrhage and other complications is higher than for singletons.
- The need for caesarean or forceps delivery is on average far greater.

- In addition to close monitoring of the babies in labour, skilled anaesthesia is required.

- Small and/or growth-retarded babies are at particular risk from the trauma of labour. This is the main reason why the risk of twins dying around birth and in the first week of life is roughly four times greater than for singletons.

- You cannot get specialist paediatric care or technical back-up at home.

Perhaps you had a home birth for your last baby, or promised yourself that you would this time, but you cannot rely on a problem-free labour and birth where twins and higher multiples are concerned. These pregnancies are by definition abnormal. Being in cosy familiar surroundings at home may make you more relaxed, so that you may feel the pain less. Admittedly you cannot change a hospital environment much, but, with proper preparation and a good relationship with the team looking after you, there are ways of feeling more in control and enjoying the birth without the risks posed by having your twins at home.

Chapter Four

YOUR NEWBORN BABIES

· *In Hospital* ·

What newborn babies look like

It is often said all babies look the same, but they don't. They may be small and wrinkled, or chubby and Churchillian; they could be hairy and will probably be covered with a greasy layer of vernix (a substance that protects them from amniotic fluid).

Your babies may not be much alike. Size can be one obvious difference. The average birth weight of twins is 2.5 kg (5 lb 8 oz), with boys being a bit heavier than girls and non-identical (DZ) twins slightly heavier than identicals. There is, however, considerable variation. Size differences are often greatest between otherwise identical twins, a fact which even some professionals do not realize.

Newborn triplets each weigh on average 1.8 kg (4 lb), but a quarter of them weigh less than 1.5 kg (3 lb 5 oz). Quads tend to weigh in at 1.4 kg (3 lb) each or less, but again this varies a great deal.

Your babies may have different-shaped bodies. One may be short and podgy while the other is long and lean. Only one thing is certain: you will love them from the start. Or will you?

· *Bonding* ·

I can honestly say that, slimy and bloody as they still were, my babies were both the most beautiful things I'd ever set eyes on.

Mothers (and their partners) are sometimes overwhelmed by love for their baby as soon as they see him. Bonding refers to what a parent feels for a young baby, an emotional tug which is a one-way process, at least at first. It probably begins in the womb with the kicking sensations and the other changes that take place in the mother's body and is reinforced by see-ing the scan or hearing a baby's heartbeat if the midwife uses a 'Doppler' machine. Falling in love with two or more babies at once can be a tall order. Rather like getting to know sever-al new people at a party, it is not always straightforward, especially if you have trouble telling them apart and little time for socializing with each one.

According to one piece of research, 71 per cent of mothers of singletons experience an immediate rush of love for their babies, but only 50 per cent of mothers of twins do. Bonding with more than one tends to be especially hard if you didn't know until delivery just how many you were having, though nowadays this is very unusual.

Soon you will discover that their temperaments or voices differ, but for now you need something more obvious to iden-tify your babies – and not just an ankle tag that you have to peer at closely. You can identify them by:

- the colour of their blankets
- a soft toy in the cot
- ribbons on the cot-handles
- dressing them differently.

If they are healthy enough to be on the ward with you, it is a good idea to keep your babies by you at all times, so that you can get to know them more quickly. The other plus is of course the security of knowing where they are and with whom. However, if you want your babies to be in the nursery at night so that you can sleep, it doesn't mean your maternal instincts are deficient.

There is believed to be a window of opportunity just after birth when bonding is most likely to take place, or at least a best time for it to happen, especially if you are physically close to your babies and breast-feed them. However, mothers feel just as much for bottle-fed or adopted babies and one can also feel deeply and passionately for a baby who is stillborn. So even if you are forcibly separated from your babies soon after birth, you can still develop the ties that bind.

What improves bonding?

Bonding is helped by seeing and holding your babies immediately after birth, but there is a variety of other things you may be able to do:

- seeing ultrasound pictures of your babies in pregnancy, especially if you are given a photo of the scan to keep
- attending parentcraft classes, with your partner if possible, particularly if these cater for multiples, so that you can form realistic expectations of your babies' first days
- meeting other parents of twins and more
- arranging some domestic help in advance
- seeking counselling during pregnancy if there are problems, for instance if you have trouble coming to terms with multiples or with an unplanned pregnancy
- considering involving the Social Services if there are likely to be great difficulties
- getting the delivery you are happy with, which may include getting rid of hangers-on in the labour ward.

Bonding with triplets, quads and more

Triplets and more may seem a blessing or a curse. A mother will often experience immense pride, but may also feel considerable trepidation. Just how is it possible to get to know and love so many babies? Can one hug these tiny individuals without harming them? (A worry fathers in particular may have.) The situation may well be made more difficult if one or more of them has to be in the SCBU (special care baby unit).

You can only do your best. One piece of research from Israel suggests that some mothers bond with their triplets or quads 'by degrees', getting acquainted with one or perhaps two at a time. If you have enlisted some help, try to arrange things so that you rotate which baby you have to yourself, to give both you and him time together.

Favourites

Parents often worry about having a favourite, although they don't always talk about it. Rest assured: this is usually a passing phase. No two people are truly identical and we shouldn't be too surprised at feeling slightly differently about our babies.

This is especially true when there are noticeable differences. There is often some favouritism early on with boy–girl pairs, or with twins of whom only one is physically attractive. Or one baby may be more placid while the other is harder to comfort. Research carried out with TAMBA also found that birth-weight differences were significant: 84 per cent of mothers of twins who expressed a preference favoured the heavier baby. Before the birth, mothers often anticipate that they will feel more tender towards the smaller twin, but (as Jane Spillman discovered in her research) this is not what usually happens.

Although there is no instant 'cure' for favouritism, nature

usually ensures that the emotions of a parent wax and wane. One of the best things you can do in such a situation is to spend a little unhurried time with each of your babies, especially the one you relate to less well. Get someone (friend, parent, partner, midwife, trainee nursery nurse – anyone you trust) to look after the other one while you attend solely to the baby for whom you feel less. Even at this early stage, you will find that being with one baby without having to think about the other gives you the chance to have one-to-one communication, something which is in short supply when you have multiples. You don't have to fall in love with the baby instantly – in fact, you probably won't. Just get to know him a little as an individual so that your feelings can develop when they are ready. (There is more about favouritism and older twins in Chapter 8.)

I called bonding a one-way process, but there is some evidence that even new babies respond to people, especially to those who seem to like them. One piece of research suggests that babies even share adult perceptions of attractiveness, preferring faces which are reasonably nice-looking. Perhaps it is worth smiling at your twins! One new mother said, 'I'd heard that babies liked happy faces better than grumpy ones, so I tried to make a big effort, even in the special care unit.'

The death of a twin either in pregnancy or soon after birth is increasingly recognized as an obstacle to bonding with the survivor. Mixed feelings are normal at this time. The pain of loss is so intimately bound up with the presence of the survivor that it makes it enormously difficult for a bond to develop. If you are bereaved in this way, try not to deny the loss. It will help to remember the dead baby, especially if you can keep some tangible evidence of his existence. This is dealt with in Chapter 14.

Fortunately, bereavement is something that relatively few parents have to go through. A more common situation is when one or more babies has to be admitted to the SCBU (special care baby unit) or NICU (neonatal intensive care unit). Albeit temporary, this enforced separation makes it harder to feel close to your babies.

In the special care baby unit (SCBU)

Once upon a time, most twins automatically went into special care if they weighed less than 2.5 kg (5^1/$_2$ lb), but this is no longer a blanket ruling. However, your babies will usually still need the specialized care of SCBU if they:

- weigh under 1.7 kg (about 3^1/$_2$ lb)
- were born before 32 weeks of pregnancy
- inhaled meconium (a baby's bowel contents) during labour
- have fits
- are jaundiced
- have a major infection or some other specific problem.

Triplets and quads, being often both small and premature, are more likely to spend some time in the SCBU. Over a quarter of triplets and nearly two-thirds of quads spend a month or more in special care, with all the difficulties that this can entail for you and the rest of the family.

Medical care

The concept of special care is simple: to reproduce as faithfully as possible the care the babies would have had in the womb. Premature babies need:

- warmth
- nourishment
- protection from infection.

Some babies need more intensive care. Breathing difficulties are common because immature lungs lack a chemical called surfactant. Without it, air enters the lung only with great effort on the part of the baby. For this reason, among others, a premature baby may need a ventilator to breathe for him. He may also need special feeding via a tube or even a vein.

Whatever treatment your babies have, their condition will be closely monitored. Using a combination of machinery and manpower, it is possible to keep a constant watch on a baby's blood pressure, heart rate, fluid balance and the amount of oxygen carried in the blood. Some parents are horrified to find that one or other baby is barely visible within an arsenal of machines and monitors. Although the concept behind special care may not be complicated, the technology used to deliver it can be daunting until you are familiar with it.

Will your babies be all right? Well, there have been huge advances in what is called neonatal (or newborn) medicine and nursing. For instance, doctors can now give surfactant, which premature lungs do not yet produce. New ventilators can now sense an infant's own weak efforts at breathing and synchronize with it. Recent developments in ultrasound mean that scans of a baby's skull can tell paediatricians what is going on inside it and help predict any risk of handicap. What this all boils down to is that you have good grounds for optimism. The survival rate for small vulnerable babies is now much improved, and fewer than ever before will have any long-term disability.

The only honest answer to the question 'Will my babies be all right?' is that it depends on their individual situation, but just look at the photos in the unit – almost every SCBU has a notice-board covered with pictures of healthy smiling children, all former patients who survived and are now enjoying life to the full.

What can a parent do in the special care unit?

If your babies are going to go to the SCBU, ask if you can touch them or hold them – even if only for a moment – before they are taken to their incubators. Early contact is valuable, but the staff may not think of it unless you mention it to them. On the other hand, there is no need to worry if you do not get a chance to hold them immediately after birth: this does not mean relationship difficulties are inevitable in the future.

Although you may not be able to cuddle your babies much once they are in the SCBU, there is still a lot you can do for them:

- Most units will offer you a Polaroid of your babies, so that even if you have no crib next to you on the postnatal ward, you will have a picture. You can ask about taking your own photos or a video as long as you do this without using a flash or getting in the way.

- As soon as you can, start spending time in the unit. If you had a caesarean in the last few hours, someone can give you a hand to visit your babies, or take you down there in a wheelchair if necessary.

- You may want to breast-feed your babies and this is often possible (by expressing milk) even when they are in special care. On the other hand, you may be surprised to learn that some premature babies don't thrive on breast milk; in these cases it is often possible to fortify your milk with a special supplement to help increase growth.

- Or you might like to help bottle-feed your babies instead. Talk to the nursing and medical staff as soon as you can about feeding. If a baby has already been started on bottles, it is possible, but more difficult, to breast-feed him later.

- Stroke your babies, if only through the 'port-holes' of the incubator. This will feel unnatural to begin with, but frequent touching is beneficial for you and your babies. You will gradually get to know each other. Babies are believed to be able to recognize a mother's touch. You will also gain confidence in handling them, which helps bonding.

- If only one of your babies is unwell, you may feel torn between the one in special care and the one on the ward – and they may be a long trek apart. You may be concerned about the welfare or safety of the one left unattended while you visit the special care unit. It is vital for mothers to have their twins close together, so ask. Perhaps you and the healthier baby can at least be moved to a ward nearer the SCBU.

- Ask if you can take the well baby with you to visit his twin. This may not mean much to him, but it often makes mothers feel better.

- If possible, get photos taken of the babies together to reinforce their twinship. This, says midwife Jane Spillman, is terribly important to mothers, especially when one baby is ill.

- Small-for-dates or prem (premature) babies may be less attractive even to their own parents (mothers often feel this though they may not like to admit it). When only one baby is unwell, nurses may encourage you to concentrate on the healthy baby, but your sicker twin needs your care and attention – and so do you. Rest assured that your well twin won't suffer as a result. If you want to be alone with the sicker one, say so. On the other hand some mothers like the companionship of a friendly nurse when they handle a very sickly baby.

- You may be afraid of developing feelings in case your baby dies, leaving you more distressed than if you had never become attached to him, but this is not borne out by the experience of parents who have been bereaved. In fact, they tend to report the opposite, and cherish whatever contact they had before they lost their child. If you have this type of worry, talk to staff on the unit. The consultant paediatrician will usually be experienced in these matters.

- Ask about your babies' treatment and get involved in their care. There may be quite a lot of day-to-day tasks you can take on, especially as your babies' health improves. Hospital policy has changed a lot – and so has the thinking on infection. Nowadays immediate family (including other children) can often spend time on special care units.

- On the unit, you may well make friends with other parents and exchange views, but don't assume that what is happening to other babies will apply to yours. Ask medical staff for information about your situation. They (or the nurses) are usually happy to explain what some of the machinery does too, all of which will reassure you.

Will my babies grow?

If your babies are small, you may wonder whether they will ever catch up. This is a tough question to answer but it needs to be addressed because so many mothers of small or prem babies want to know, and yet are afraid to ask because they anticipate a disheartening reply.

Size does seem to be important. It is particularly important to parents of multiples when only one baby is small because the difference between a tiny scrap of an infant and his bouncing sibling of the same age is all too obvious – to themselves and anyone they come into contact with.

As a rule, small babies grow well if they are small only because they were born too soon. The more premature they are, the longer they take to catch up, so if your babies are both (or all) small because they arrived two months prematurely, you can expect the early disparity to vanish over the next couple of years.

There are a few exceptions, for instance when the placenta functions less than adequately. If a baby happens to be unduly small for the length of time spent in the womb, he may not catch up. A baby very much smaller than her twin

(or her co-triplets) may therefore remain petite. This is especially true when a baby faces a great many medical problems
as a newborn.

Babies do confound the issue by coming in various shapes
and sizes, but you can get a rough idea of a baby's potential
for growth from his length. If he is underweight for the age at
which he was born but is a good length, he may make up his
weight easily, often within a few weeks of birth.

When will they come home?

It is hard to say exactly when this will happen, apart from
the obvious answer 'When they are ready'. This may be ages
after (or even long before) you are ready for them. Whenever
they come home, however, this is the next phase of the
biggest adventure of your life.

The smaller or more premature your babies are, the likelier
it is that you will have to leave one of them in hospital when
you are sent home. Nevertheless, many units will do their best
to keep both babies together instead of creating chaos for you
by discharging them at different times. Whether this is possible depends on the facilities at that particular hospital and,
unfortunately, their services are likely to be fully stretched.

Sometimes only one baby is in special care; occasionally
babies are even in different hospitals. This is far from ideal
from the parent's point of view, but sometimes it cannot be
helped, for instance with higher-order multiples. For the
parent and the rest of the family, it creates unwelcome
differences between the babies right from the start. It feels
wrong, somehow, because this is a time when normally you
would all be together as a family. Just spending time with an
absent baby can also create a number of practical problems.

- Visit as much as possible. The baby in a remote hospital is
  still part of the family and needs to take his place in it as
  soon as he can.

- Breast-feeding, even if only partial, can help.

- Talk about your baby to any friends or relatives who cannot visit him.

- You may have difficulty bonding with the sickest baby, so don't expect to feel instant love for him.

Some mothers find that having one baby home at a time is far easier and gives them a chance to get adjusted to each one separately.

> Yes, it was very hard having each of my triplets discharged from hospital at different times, but I don't know how I would have managed had they all come home together, needing three-hourly feeds.

Chapter Five

FEEDING AND OTHER PRACTICALITIES

When they have their first scan, many women give up the idea of breast-feeding because they think it is impossible to breast-feed two or more babies. It is, in fact, perfectly feasible and mothers have successfully breast-fed twins for centuries, even if some professionals today still don't realize it.

The size of your breasts does not determine whether or not you will succeed at breast-feeding. One mother (who takes a 36A bra) recalls how hurt she felt when told by the midwife, inaccurately as it turned out, that she would never have enough milk.

Breast-feeding twins is, however, more demanding than with a singleton and you need to find out as much as you can about it, which is where TAMBA can help. Then make up your own mind how you want to feed your babies. Try to be honest with yourself and, whatever you decide, don't feel guilty or pressurized. This is easier said than done, especially if it is your first pregnancy, but you need to be at ease with your decision and with your body. It is a myth that you can bond with your baby only if you breast-feed him. On the contrary, if you are unhappy about breast-feeding you may resent it and bond less well with your babies.

Although you may be advised to put your babies to the breast immediately after birth to get breast-feeding established, it is not essential, so there is no need to be despondent if you don't get a chance to do this. Also, don't rely too much on any previous experience of breast-feeding. If this is your second pregnancy, you may find that the milk flows more easily than it did the first time.

In favour of breast-feeding

- The perfect food for babies in terms of suitability, breast milk also comes ready prepared and at the right temperature.

- Breast milk contains antibodies which protect against infection. It is especially beneficial in the first three or four months, before a baby produces his own antibodies.

- Because it is a supply-and-demand arrangement, you are unlikely to overfeed.

- Breast milk protects against severe gastro-enteritis, partly because of the antibodies it contains and partly because it requires no preparation.

- Breast-fed babies are thought to suffer less eczema and/or asthma (this is not proven, however).

- Breast-feeding brings you physically (and possibly emotionally) closer to your babies. As a result your babies may be more satisfied, though sadly there are no guarantees.

- Breast-feeding helps the womb contract back to its normal size and (because it burns calories) can also help you regain your figure. The jury is still out as to whether it protects against breast cancer in later life.

- It is cheaper than bottle-feeding, though you will have to eat and drink more.

- Breast-fed babies need less 'winding'.

- Full breast-feeding (i.e. without any bottle-feeding) offers some protection against pregnancy, but don't bank on it, especially since mothers of multiples tend to be more fertile.

- Breast-feeding feels nice. For some women it is an intensely sexual experience.

In favour of bottle-feeding

- Someone else can easily feed your babies. This gives others (your partner, for example) a greater chance to be involved in their care and it gives you an opportunity to do other things, such as sleep, go back to work, shop, or look after your other children.

- You don't get sore nipples.

- You can still cuddle your babies and hold them close.

- You know how much nourishment they are getting. On average, every 24 hours a baby needs 2–3 fl oz of formula milk for each pound he weighs (100–170 ml per kg). This is just a rough guide; babies vary.

- Since you don't have to bare your breasts several times a day and you don't leak (after the first few days), you can wear what you want.

- You can feed your babies wherever you like (in winter, breast-feeding can be inconvenient, if not downright cold).

- Bottle-feeding demands special equipment and preparation (and greater cost) but is less taxing physically. It's possible that you will return to your normal mental state more quickly; you will sweat less at night, too.

- Your babies may sleep through the night more soundly. A breast-fed baby could be waking at night not just for a feed, but for a 'human dummy' as well, which may perpetuate the habit.

- Older siblings may be less jealous.

All in all, it is a personal decision and a lot depends on you and your life-style. If you are still unsure, try talking to an expert, for instance from TAMBA, La Leche League or the NCT. A mother of twins can breast-feed if she sets her mind to it. Other things being equal – and if you are in reasonable health yourself – you might like to start by breast-feeding. You can always change to bottles later, but once babies start sucking from an artificial teat it can be harder to win them over to the breast.

· *Breast-Feeding Twins* ·

The principles of nutrition, nipple care and latching on are the same with twins as with a single baby and your midwife, antenatal clinic or breast-feeding counsellor can give you plenty of general information. This section concentrates on areas which are of special interest to the mothers of twins.

A routine is vital when you have more than one baby and you will want to get into one as early as possible. All the same, it is usual to begin by feeding new babies on demand: whenever they seem hungry. This is important because you build up a supply of milk based on how much the babies suckle. If your twins are very small or premature, you may be advised to feed them every two or three hours, regardless of whether or not they are hungry.

Because feeding would otherwise take up the whole day, it is normal to feed both babies simultaneously unless there is a good reason not to. If one wakes for a feed, rouse the other one. He may not take much at this feed, but with luck the babies will eventually synchronize. The other advantage of feeding both at the same time is that the other breast will not leak uselessly, as it often does when feeding a singleton. You may want to feed your babies separately if they are of very different sizes and hence have different nutritional needs.

Apart from this, the most obvious difference when breast-feeding twins is positioning. Some mothers have them in the same position as a single baby (as shown in the diagram), but this gives no control over their bodies; they may also kick each other throughout the feed.

The more popular position for twins is the 'football' hold shown. This allows you to control their bodies a bit, you are cuddling them more and their legs don't get in the way.

Some mothers compromise and have their babies more or less parallel during feeds, which can work well. As you will find for yourself, there are other possibilities too.

Your own comfort is crucially important. You are likely to be feeding for several hours a day, which puts immense strain on your neck, shoulders and back. Your back needs to be supported and your babies raised to nipple level. Many mothers find a large V-shaped or triangular cushion essential,

Some positions for breast-feeding twins

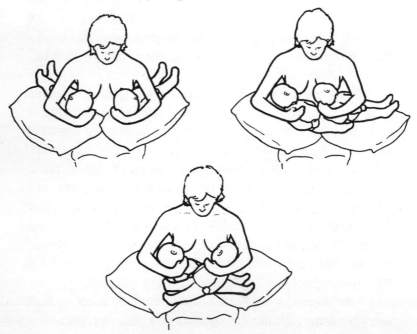

but other cushions or pillows will work as long as the whole arrangement is secure.

A good place to feed twins is on a sofa or bed. Single beds are usually too narrow to accommodate you, babies and cushions without something vital falling off; this is a common difficulty in hospital. You may be better off sitting sideways on, but make sure your back is supported. What seems comfortable to begin with can change over the next twenty minutes or half hour, especially if one or other baby comes off the nipple and has to be helped to latch on again.

Getting and keeping the babies securely latched on is the main difficulty to begin with and you may feel you don't have enough arms. While you are still in hospital, get a midwife to stay with you throughout the feed, to give you a hand in case one baby comes off the nipple in mid-feed.

Premature babies tend to suck less well, especially if born before 34 weeks or so. Small babies can also be hard to feed if you have big breasts which seem to engulf them. The opposite is not easy either: if you have smallish breasts and fairly big babies it can be awkward to get comfortable particularly if the babies take it into their heads to move during the feed.

Once you've got the hang of it, though, you will become adept at managing on your own. You will find that, compared with friends who breast-feed only one baby, there is a snag: a lot of so called maternity and nursing clothes are unsuitable. Of what use is just one limited opening down the front? It is sometimes possible to find night-dresses with two slits, one over each breast. With other garments you may as well just choose a top you can unbutton completely or lift up. Some mothers do not like exposing themselves to this extent, but others couldn't care less.

Some mothers swap breasts at each feed, while others keep one breast for each baby. Since babies don't always need the same amount of nourishment, this can result in temporary lop-sidedness. If your babies are very different in weight you may prefer to alternate breasts.

For how long should you feed at each session? The usual answer is however long the babies want. However, they may want to go on sucking for comfort long after they have technically been fed and you could end up with sore nipples, which will put you off the whole thing. In general, fair-skinned women can stand less sucking. It is best to feed as often as the babies seem to want, but if you cannot manage to let them suck for as long as they want, rest assured that five to ten minutes at the breast per feed will usually drain most of the milk.

You can always express milk if your breasts are engorged, or you want someone else to feed for you, perhaps if your babies are in the special care unit. If you express milk more than just occasionally, a hand-operated breast pump will not be enough; you will need an electrical one. You can hire this from the NCT, or ask the hospital. Most women who have tried one say the machine makes them feel like a cow, but they often add 'So what?'

In the weeks and months that you are breast-feeding, make sure you have plenty to drink. Guinness is the traditional recommendation, although it is probably no better or worse than other calorific fluids. A small amount of alcohol may help to relax you but don't overdo it: an excess could be harmful to your babies. Make sure you eat enough, too, especially protein and carbohydrate. Nature has a way of fixing things and the best plan is just to eat when you are hungry. Now is not the time to diet.

You may want to breast-feed for just a few weeks, or for many months. Whatever you can manage will probably benefit the babies and many mothers have successfully fed their twins exclusively on breast milk till the end of the first year. If you are happy with it, and the babies are thriving, there is no reason why you shouldn't too. Alternatively, you may want to stop when they start solids at four to five months. This is often a time when their requirements increase anyway, so you may find it something of a struggle to keep breast-feeding. A few mothers point out that it is messy too, from the solids the babies have managed to smear on to themselves – and then on to you.

There may be other times when you want to top up with a bottle of formula milk, which is known as complementary feeding. Mixing breast and bottle works well for some and can enable a mother to breast-feed when she would otherwise have given up. The snag with bottles – apart from having to prepare them – is that a baby then sucks less from the breast, decreasing the milk supply. If you are going to offer bottles as well, make sure you do so just after a breast-feed, not before.

If you have a partner, his support is vital to breast-feeding twins successfully. At first you may simply need help in getting set up and moral support if things aren't going smoothly, but later on, when you are skilled at it, breast-feeding multiples is still a commitment. It is time-consuming and you will need to rest more than if you only had one baby. Meanwhile, the number of chores you have to do is at least double that for a singleton.

Various sources can give you advice on breast-feeding and a visit to another mother who is breast-feeding twins can be very helpful. However, not all professionals believe it can be done. Unless you tell your GP, he or she may not realize that you have succeeded. Many drugs pass into breast milk, so remind your doctor that you are breast-feeding if you are prescribed anything or recommended to take any medication.

Breast-Feeding Triplets

One obvious problem here is that a woman has a maximum of only two breasts. However, it is possible to breast-feed triplets, and is a good idea, if you feel so inclined. You will be even shorter of time, but breast-feeding gives you a chance to cuddle up to your babies, and, being generally smaller and more premature than twins, triplets (and more) can benefit even more from the goodness of breast milk. The down side is:

- your babies are more likely to be in the SCBU
- they may not suck well if they are very premature.

Breast-feeding three is thoroughly exhausting, but many women have successfully managed it – and enjoyed it – for as long as six months or more. TAMBA Supertwins Group can put you in touch with mothers who are happy to share their experiences and pass on practical advice. This is especially useful if you've come into contact with midwives or other professionals who are convinced it cannot be done.

Your choice lies between

- breast-feeding one or two babies and bottle-feeding the other(s), perhaps on a rota basis so that every 24 hours all get breast-feeds and all get bottles
- breast-feeding two and giving your expressed milk to the third
- breast-feeding all three at different times (very time-consuming).

You can use the positions and principles described above for breast-feeding twins. If you have a helper, he or she can take the third baby. Or you may be able to position him safely near you, even perched atop your V-shaped pillow.

To make a go of breast-feeding triplets, you really have to put your own health first. This means rest, healthy food and plenty to drink have to be a priority. You should then be able to produce enough milk. If you are not sure you are succeeding in nourishing three, weigh your babies more often, say twice a week. With triplets, your health visitor should be happy to come to your home to weigh the babies. If she doesn't offer, ask. Better still, insist.

· *Bottle-Feeding Twins* · *or More*

Although bottles may seem an easier option, it is hard to get close to two or more babies and keep the bottles in the right position, let alone rub your nose if it happens to get itchy during a feed, for example. Again, the general principles are the same as for bottle-feeding any baby, though there are a few differences.

Position

Finding the right position depends to a great extent on how big your babies are. Using cushions to support your arms, you will probably find it best to hold a bottle in each hand and have a baby on either side of you, either:

- alongside each of your legs
- with a head resting on each of your thighs
- or with a baby on each arm (you need fairly supple wrists for this).

You could also prop the babies up side by side and hold their bottles rather than them, but then you won't be physically close to them.

With practice, you will soon settle on one position – or several – which you find most convenient. If there is another adult about, you can each feed a baby like a singleton. However short of arms you are, never leave a baby propped up with a bottle unsupervised.

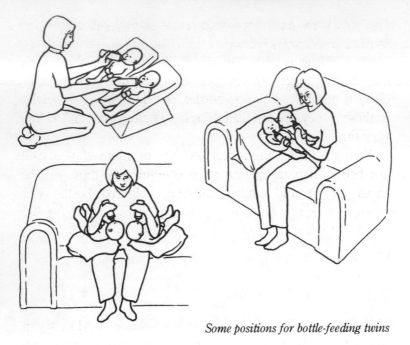

Some positions for bottle-feeding twins

Timing

As with breast-feeding, your aim is to get into a regular routine as soon as you can, but you generally need to start off by feeding on demand. It is often best to feed twins simultaneously, waking the one who is not hungry yet. The one you've woken may not take as much at this feed as the one who's vociferously requesting his bottle, but it all works out after a while. However, if they are of very different weights, you risk overfeeding one of them, and you may be better off catering to their individual needs: feeding them separately from the start even though it takes longer.

Preparing feeds

Preparing feeds up to 24 hours in advance is fine if you have enough bottles – and space in the fridge. As an alternative to storing individual bottles, you could use large measuring jugs full of formula. This needs to be stirred before pouring from it; use a sterile spoon.

Don't forget to shake bottles before you give them. You may be able to get by with one sterilizing unit at first, especially if you have half-size bottles, but don't invest specially in these – they are not useful for long unless your babies are very tiny.

Two sterilizing units (borrow one or more if you can) are better than using one huge container as they will be easier to lift and empty. Different coloured bottles (for example, blue and red caps) are handy so you can remember which baby had what, particularly if you have to break off mid-feed.

Reheating cold bottles

Many babies will accept cold bottles. However, cold milk can cool a young baby down too much. It is better to heat it up first, but milk which is too hot is very dangerous. It can cause the lining of the back of the throat to swell up, which can asphyxiate and even kill a baby. A microwave oven may seem a good method for reheating bottles, especially when preparing two or more at a time, but there is a risk of it creating hot spots in the milk. Instead you can use a bottle warmer, or rather two, or just a bowl of hot water.

Another useful tip for reheating cold bottles is to deliberately make up the formula with insufficient water and add hot later when you want it. For instance, if your babies need 180 mls (6 fl oz), make bottles up in advance with enough scoops of powder for this amount, but only 120 mls (4 fl oz) of water, and leave them in the fridge. Just before you give the feed, add the remaining quantity of freshly boiled (hot) water. A little practice will enable you to get the proportions right. Of course, never give (or let anyone else give) formula which is too concentrated. If someone else will be feeding, the bottles should be carefully labelled to show that top-up is needed.

Whatever means you use for preparing bottle-feeds, you must still test the temperature every time. The traditional way is to sprinkle a few drops on to the inside of your wrist.

· *Nappies* ·

Disposable or terry?

Disposable nappies are a great boon and are now made to fit almost all shapes and sizes of bottoms. Most mothers of twins go for disposables, but this depends on you and your life-style. Terries aren't necessarily ecologically sounder since they have to be washed, using electricity and detergent, and terries are no better or worse for nappy rash than disposable nappies. Once you've bought them, they work out a little cheaper, but obviously they are going to be more time-consuming – a vital consideration with two or more babies.

If you go for terries, you will need to splash out on about three dozen for twins. It sounds a lot, but some will be in soak. Use two nappy buckets if necessary rather than a single huge one which can be back-breaking to handle when full.

If you decide to take the disposable route, consider frequenting a cash and carry to get a better price, or get nappies delivered to save time and energy. Some firms deliver for very little extra and it can make life a lot easier. They may also stock other supplies such as formula or baby toiletries.

When to change?

Before a feed would seem handy, in case the babies doze off while feeding, but this can delay – noisily – a hungry baby's feed. Besides, feeding tends to fill a nappy (the official term is the gastro-colic reflex) so all in all it is best to change a nappy after a feed unless it was already dirty or soaking wet. Keep nappy-changing gear both upstairs and downstairs to save you running up and down too many times.

· *Bathing* ·

You don't have to bath your twins every day. It can of course be a form of playtime for them and you, but there are less tiring ways of playing together. Besides, some babies hate baths and are very vocal about letting you know it.

Newborn babies mainly get dirty at each end, so just keep their faces and nappy areas clean on a daily basis. Use warm water and cotton wool. You need only bath each baby on alternate days, unless you want and can do it more often. (Incidentally, there is no need to change the water for each baby unless the first one opens his bowels in it, but that rarely happens). To save your back, use a stand for the bath, and don't carry around full baby baths unnecessarily.

· *Avenues of Help* ·

If you didn't know it already, by the time you've read this far you will have some idea of how busy you will be with more than one new baby. Apart from feeding and changing, there is bathing, washing, shopping, not to mention the rest of life . . . . You need help. If this is your first pregnancy, you may be all at sea. If you already have children you will have even more to do.

Perhaps you've already got something organized, or made tentative enquiries, but most expectant mothers wait until after the birth, by which time they are surrounded by demanding babies and find it more difficult to make sensible arrangements.

What you need depends on your circumstances. Who else is there around? Do you have other children? Will you be at work? Can you afford paid help? Have you a spare room?

The ideal helper is practical, willing, and reliable, not just someone who pops round every so often for cups of tea and coos over your little bundles.

- Your partner is the most obvious source of help (and moral support) in the first few days at home, especially if he can negotiate time off work. This can be a very special time, when you can get to know your babies together and bond more closely as a couple, as well as getting on with chores. Even men who profess not to know one extremity of a baby from the other can turn out to be willing helpers.

- Grandparents who live nearby can be worth their weight in gold. They will adore the grandchildren and boast about 'their' twins or triplets. However, if you have waited years to start your family, your parents may be elderly and less fit. They may also be full of old-fashioned ideas; even up-to-date suggestions may not be much use if they apply only to singletons. You have to accentuate the positive aspects of relationships with grandparents and accept their unique contribution, while learning where to draw the line.

- Neighbours and friends are useful if they have time they can reliably spare. The trouble here is that they are often delighted to admire the babies but cannot make a regular commitment. If you have an acquaintance who can – or who has a teenaged son or daughter who is willing – consider paying them to put the arrangement on a business-like footing.

- Volunteers from your local church or other local groups may be happy to help. Or you could contact Home-Start, a charity which has local networks of trained volunteers who help young families in their own home. Your health visitor, GP or midwife may also have ideas. However, some professionals are still underinformed about the needs of multiples and are less than helpful.

On the whole, there is little support for new mothers of multiples, as research for TAMBA confirms. Unless there are compelling social reasons, Social Services have little to offer mothers of twins or triplets, but may be able to assist those with quads or quins. If you are offered a home help, establish what she will do and when. It is pointless being told you can have two hours of home help a week, without knowing when those two hours will be; this sometimes happens.

Paid help

This includes:

- Maternity nurses: highly skilled (and highly paid) help for the first few weeks.

- Nannies: either untrained or fully qualified; can be daily or live-in. A qualified daily nanny is the most expensive, and an untrained – but experienced – person may be preferable, especially as she will often be prepared to do more housework (negotiate at interview, not later on). As a mother of twins, you do not usually want someone to be with the babies, leaving you with all the chores.

- Mother's helps: do not usually have sole charge of the children and are willing to do housework.

- *Au pairs*: very variable in skills and attitude. They should not usually be expected to cope on their own with very young babies, but can still be helpful if you have the space.

Help at night is a godsend, especially in the first three months, but it is worth remembering that a baby's cries often wake only the mother, not the nanny!

One promising source of part-time help is a local college NNEB (Nursery Nurse Education Board) course. A student nanny on this course is often only too pleased to be involved with twins or triplets in her final year and may be able to manage as much as a day a week for up to a year.

Whatever kind of help you arrange, and whether or not she lives in with you for the time being, as a parent you have to learn to make some space in your lives for her. This bit can take getting used to.

> We couldn't have managed without Fran [*au pair*], but we really wished we didn't need her. It was my first pregnancy and we had intended to spend the first days and weeks as a family to enjoy that special time together. However, since our baby turned out to be triplets, this became an impossible dream.

· *Crying* ·

Your babies may not cry much. Many don't, though mine certainly did. Fortunately, newborn twins don't often set each other off crying, though it seems like it because they have similar needs at similar times. This is perhaps the essence of the problem of bringing up multiples. They will obviously cry together when they are hungry, tired or colicky at the same time. You will learn to anticipate some of their wants, which is where a routine really comes into its own. On the other hand, some mothers have found that when one baby is screaming for something, the other one is mercifully quiet.

Why are they crying?

Crying in stereo puts appalling pressure on a parent. What should you do first? Why are they crying, anyway? It could be:

- hunger – you will soon learn to distinguish this cry from the way it builds up in pitch
- discomfort or pain
- boredom – especially after four weeks of age
- a dirty nappy – possibly, though research shows that a baby is often satisfied if his dirty nappy is removed and then replaced without changing. (However, do change nappies often, if only to prevent rashes.)

Are they ill? You should suspect this if one or other baby

- is drowsy
- is unusually fractious or awkward
- is off his feed
- has a dry nappy when you would expect it to be wet (a sign of dehydration)
- has loose stools
- is snuffly
- has noisy or laboured breathing.

If any of these applies, or if you are worried, check with your GP or health visitor without delay. Inevitably, there will be a false alarm or two, but most family doctors are happy to help as they know that new parents are anxious; most GPs are parents too. If, however, your doctor is not all that interested in young families (after all, everyone has different areas of expertise), consider changing your GP.

In time, you will learn to trust your instincts and will recognize what your babies need when they are crying. Meanwhile, watch out for the danger signs mentioned. A digital thermometer, used under the baby's arm, can help you decide when an infant is ill. Although not infallible, it is more accurate than a heat-sensitive strip held on to the forehead.

Colic

Regular crying, particularly in the evenings, can be colic, a poorly understood condition which usually starts at two weeks of age and disappears at three months. It is also known as 'evening colic' and 'three-month colic'. It is thought that there may be a link between colic and milk intolerance, so in severe cases it may be worth changing your babies to a soya-based feed. Talk to your doctor first about this and other possible remedies. Otherwise, just cuddle and comfort your colicky baby. Babies should not be put to sleep on their fronts, but holding him on his stomach, for instance draped over your forearm, may relieve your baby's discomfort. However, two colicky babies could soon wear out your arms and your patience.

Coping with crying babies

If your babies are crying but you know they are not hungry, thirsty, bored or ill, you must get through this time as best you can. Fortunately, someone other than their mother usually finds it easier. One good way of defusing the situation is to collar someone into looking after the babies while you go and sit (or lie) down quietly out of earshot for half an hour.

You can also try playing them music – Mozart and Simon and Garfunkel are popular with many babies – or a tape of 'womb noises', available in shops. The sound of a vacuum cleaner also soothes some crying babies.

Putting on some music and leaving the room can work wonders for all of you, but it requires a mother with an iron will. And first you have to make sure your babies won't come to any harm unsupervised.

Many mothers cope with crying twins by bundling them into the pram and wheeling them round the block. Alternatively, you could try a drive in the car. If this does the trick, you can stop and read a book, or else come home and try to get them back in the house without waking them up.

Dummies

With twins or more, the babies have to wait about a great deal while you are changing, dressing or bathing the other(s). Here dummies can be a real boon. There are fears that dummies may interfere with the development of teeth or speech, but if you use them only occasionally problems shouldn't arise. Besides, a baby usually gives up his dummy when he no longer needs it. It helps if you:

- restrict a dummy to indoor use only
- do not let a baby who can walk use one
- use the dummy not as a toy but as an aid to sanity
- stop offering one if the baby doesn't seek it.

Do keep dummies clean and sterilize them often (a spare set is a good idea). Never keep a dummy on a ribbon around a baby's neck: he shouldn't need a dummy constantly and, more importantly, there is a risk of him strangling.

Where to turn

If you have trouble coping with crying babies, don't be ashamed of asking for help. After all, many mothers of singletons need to and the burdens on you are that much greater. Sharing your frustrations and difficulties, especially when your babies are very demanding, is not a sign of weakness, nor does it imply that you are deficient as a parent. TAMBA Twinline (see page 343) offers support and advice to families of multiples, given by trained volunteers who are themselves parents of twins, triplets or more. Help is available in the evening and at weekends, times of greatest need, yet when professionals are often most difficult to contact.

· *Postnatal Depression* ·

Whatever happened to the image of a joyous family, with you, the serenely competent mother, doubly happy and glowing with pride? Well, that picture may well be right part of the time, but nobody is superlatively happy all the time. Some mothers find, despite their best efforts, that their pleasures are clouded and their lives dimmed to a greater or lesser extent by postnatal depression.

In its various forms, postnatal depression affects roughly 10 per cent of new mothers. Because of the greater emotional, physical and financial burdens, it is not very surprising that it is slightly more common in mothers of twins and more, at least in relatively mild forms. Over a twelve-year period, Australian research found mothers of twins to be both more anxious and more depressed postnatally than women with singletons.

Several British studies also confirm that mothers of twins suffer more from fatigue, anxiety and emotional distress. Sometimes depression persists long after babyhood. Research shows that, compared with mothers of singletons, a slightly higher proportion of mothers with five-year-old twins are depressed. In fact, depression is more common in these mothers than in those who have closely spaced single children. Mothers one of whose twins has died are, not surprisingly, especially prone to depression.

Symptoms and diagnosis

None of this means that you will inevitably become depressed, only that you should be aware of the possibility and seek the right help early on if you develop any of the symptoms, such as:

- crying more than usual
- feeling hopeless/despairing
- being unable to laugh or enjoy yourself
- becoming very introspective
- indecisiveness
- panic
- excessive guilt
- poor appetite (or, conversely, comfort-eating)
- sleeping badly (even when the babies are quiet).

Some women with postnatal depression suffer only mildly, while for others it is a major obstacle to normal life. Untreated, it can have widespread consequences, including marital problems and even child abuse. That's why it's worth taking seriously.

Unfortunately it is sometimes hard for a woman or her family to get her symptoms recognized for what they are. Tears, anxiety and indecision can be part of early life with a new baby anyway (the so-called 'three-day blues'). Professionals do not always appreciate when a woman is sliding into depression. Many doctors will assume that all is well if you don't speak up, or if you make light of your symptoms.

Some mothers do not articulate their negative feelings, afraid perhaps of being thought incapable of coping, or they simply do not mention them to the GP early enough.

> It was towards the end of the consultation when I began to feel comfortable enough to tell the doctor how I felt (including the fact that actually I didn't need the Pill she'd just pre-scribed because I doubted I'd ever want sex again). But by then I'd got up and the doctor seemed to have mentally switched into a different gear. As far as she was concerned the consultation was over. It was another two weeks before I got around to telling her what I was going through.

In an attempt to spot postnatal depression sooner, especially in its milder forms, you may be asked by your midwife or GP to complete a short questionnaire at about six weeks after birth. The ten items of the Edinburgh Questionnaire ask a mother to assess how she has felt in the last seven days. It includes such items as: 'I have blamed myself unnecessarily when things went wrong.' Using the questionnaire has not yet become routine, but so far it seems a promising way of identifying the needs of some women who would not otherwise have made their feelings known.

Causes

It is not certain what exactly brings on postnatal depression, but there are various theories. Some experts believe that, since pregnancy and labour are a time of enormous hormonal upheaval, it might be due to hormone deficiency, either of progesterone, or (according to a more recent theory) oestrogen. Proponents of each of these schools of thought have claimed success in treating depression with hormones, but not every woman responds. Besides, the hormone theories hardly explain why new fathers can also have typical postnatal depression, as more than one piece of reseach has shown!

It is likely that the acute mood swings (three-day blues) soon after birth are related to wild hormonal fluctuations, but there is less certainty about longer-term symptoms. Postnatal depression may be an accentuated reaction to the stresses of new parenthood, of which there are plenty, especially when bearing two or more babies at a time. Some of the issues researchers have identified are:

• the shock of being pregnant with more than one
• increased physical and emotional burden of multiple pregnancy
• a high level of medical intervention

- practical difficulties in caring for the new babies
- sheer exhaustion
- worry about the babies' health
- problems in bonding
- lack of support or understanding from family and friends
- siblings' reactions to the new babies
- financial worries
- isolation in the home.

Treatment

There are a number of ways of tackling postnatal depression, depending on its severity. Sometimes all a mother needs is solid support, both practical and emotional. This can come from family and helpers, and/or from talking things over on a regular basis with a friendly health visitor, GP, midwife, or another experienced mother of twins.

A few women need more than this, with formal help from a counsellor, psychiatrist, psychologist or psychotherapist. Your GP can arrange for further help.

Anti-depressants can be very useful in some cases, and – contrary to popular perception they are not habit-forming, unlike sedatives and sleeping pills. They don't work instantly, but have been known to help when nothing else seems to work. Perhaps this is because depression has a biochemical element. The newer anti-depressants generally cause less drowsiness and other side-effects, but the older types are thought to be safer if you are breast-feeding.

Some women seem to respond to oestrogens in the form of HRT (hormone replacement therapy). Patches in particular seem to be useful, according to some experts, but how useful hormones are in most cases of postnatal depression remains to be seen.

Fathers may need to have their own feelings recognized, and to have time and support to get adjusted to their new role.

Making things easier

It is not always possible to prevent postnatal depression, but positive improvements can be made on a number of fronts to ease the first hectic few weeks with your new babies:

1   Get into a routine as soon as you can. Mothers of single-tons can afford a somewhat lax happy-go-lucky attitude to feeding, bathing and sleeping – they have so much less to do than you! When asked to give just one piece of advice, mothers of twins often say: 'Get yourself organized.' And that means accepting all useful offers of help.

2   Prioritize ruthlessly. You may have washed the net cur-tains on a weekly basis before or ironed tea-towels. Those days are gone. Housework should be pruned to the basic minimum required to maintain hygiene; anything more is an optional extra. Use your spare time for something important: yourself and your immediate family.

3   Keep your own health up to par and try to get enough food, vitamins and rest. Don't forget your postnatal exercises. YOU come first since so many others now depend totally on you.

4   Team up with other mothers of twins who understand your situation and can give you much-needed support. Friends with only one baby won't understand what you have to contend with. Contact TAMBA or your local Twins Group.

5   Learn to control or release stress. Mental and physical tension often go hand in hand and it is worth learning a method of physical relaxation to help you let go. You can use a relaxation technique learnt in antenatal class-

es, or learn a new one from a video, audio cassette, book or relaxation teacher. Go to your public library or contact the Relaxation for Living Trust (see page 345).

6   Schedule a little 'me time' to do things you enjoy. This may only be a few minutes a day spent listening to music, but it is important to have some time for yourself and also for you and your partner as a couple.

7   Pre-empt guilt. A lot of advice new mothers receive is undoubtedly well meant but turns out to be either useless or else impossible to follow. You do not have to take it all to heart, nor do you have to strive to be perfect. Being a 'good-enough' parent is plenty.

8   Take steps to avoid isolation. It will be harder for you to get out and about and your pre-twins life may seem a distant and unreal experience, but soon you will want to keep in touch with friends, workmates and so on. If you cannot get out to see people, use the phone.

9   Everything may be rosy for you, but if not, or if you are having trouble coping, talk to someone. See your GP or health visitor and explain why things are becoming too much. It is not an admission of defeat, but the first step on the road to improvement.

Chapter Six

SURVIVING THE FIRST YEAR

How do mothers of singletons manage to fill their day?

It is natural that you should feel enormous pride in your babies and, besides, doesn't everyone keep saying how lucky you are to have twins? But at the end of the day any parent has only two arms and one spine and the end of the day is often when they ache most. Mothers of multiples soon find that, although they get lots of admiring glances and appreciative remarks, there are few offers of practical help. Elizabeth Bryan tells of one mother of triplets who, fed up with the intrusive questions of passers-by, put a sign on the pram saying 'donations welcome'.

Babies usually learn to walk around the age of twelve months. Because they are growing fast yet are still very dependent physically on you, the first year brings huge logistic difficulties. Obviously the more willing hands there are, the easier life is, but not everyone has willing and able grandparents or can afford paid help. Research confirms the suspicion that mothers of twins get out of the house much less often than mothers of singletons.

At home there is so much to do, as well. Studies show that a mother of twins can spend nearly twice as long on tasks related to the babies, thus halving the time spent directly with them. If you want to work out the time left for each of twins, halve that again: each twin gets about a quarter of the attention a singleton has. So when can you find time to relate to your babies and enjoy them?

· *Getting out of the House* ·

Even the simplest outing can become a real palaver when you have to get two or more babies ready at the same time, not to mention getting yourself presentable. Just when they've been fed, changed, dressed and popped into their buggy (along with nappy-changing gear and the next feed), and you have your hand on the front door to open it, you suddenly notice that one of them has a smelly nappy. You get him out and change him again, by which time his twin is screaming with impatience. It is important not to get discouraged as a little forward planning can work wonders.

> I got it down to such a fine art that my friends would marvel. How was it that I managed to mobilize my two faster than they did their singletons?

Buggies and prams

A double pram will last most of the first year and possibly well into the second, depending on your life-style. By the age of four months, however, most babies can go into a buggy, though again this depends on your routine and to some extent on the weather. Most mothers favour a side-by-side buggy so that the twins can see each other. Get a good, solid buggy, that conforms to British Standards and one that is preferably new. It will have to last you longer and will work much harder than buggies used for siblings of different ages. Before you buy, check the width (the crucial comparison is with the width of your front door or porch), weight, folding qualities and handle height of the models you are interested

in. Try getting one with a rain-hood that can stay on even
when you fold the buggy. If you are not sure exactly what
you want, you could hire one first.

Triple buggies can also be side-by-side (here, width gets
even greater and you have to consider shop entrances) or
have one seat in front. You could make do, for a while anyway, with a double buggy and a sling for one baby.

Cars

You still need a buggy even if you drive everywhere. How
can you carry both babies to your car and still open the car
door? It is much safer to put them both in their buggy for the
30 metres or whatever to the car than to take them out of the
house one by one.

If you have a choice of car at this time, you will find a four-
door model easier on yourself. Or this may be the moment
you are forced to consider something bigger, like a minibus
or people-carrier (MPV).

In the front of a car, a child under three must be in an
appropriate seat or restraint for his size. Rear-facing seats are
usually suitable for babies weighing up to 13 kg ($28^{1}/2$ lb).
Don't use these in the front if you have a passenger airbag.
You may prefer to hire rear-facing seats initially, then install
traditional forward-facing child seats which are suitable from
9 kg (20 lb) upwards and will last throughout toddlerhood.

Public transport

Although trains and undergrounds may not be too awful
with a buggy, buses are often impossible for a mother of multiples on her own. You can sometimes manage twins in two
slings, or one in a sling and the other in a buggy, but soon
your back will let you know it is too much. If you have any
choice in the matter, minimize these trips and take another
adult with you when you must go by bus.

Shopping

When the babies are in a pram or buggy, it is usually a question of going round the supermarket with it, but once the babies sit up well unaided, you may be able to get them into the child seat of a trolley. Always use a harness. In most supermarkets, you will need two trolleys, one for each twin. Push one and pull the other. Mothers of triplets or more suggest leaving at least one baby at home with someone rather than attempt shopping trips *en famille*.

Making outings easier

- Keep the nappy-changing bag always ready by the front door.
- Take toys along to allay boredom. Attaching toys to the buggy avoids too many losses. A couple of extra toys hidden away in a bag will prove useful if your outing is longer than planned.
- If bottle-feeding, have feeds ready in the fridge so that you don't come home with two starving babies and find nothing to give them.
- An extra feed in the changing bag is a good idea too.

Clinic visits

Mothers of twins and triplets tend not to weigh their babies as much as those with singletons, not because they need it less, but because it is such an ordeal getting to the clinic. Transporting them there, undressing them, dressing them again and maybe consoling them after a jab can all seem too much.

- Health visitors may not have experience of multiples, so tell yours how she can help in practical ways. Perhaps she can hold one of the babies for you, or arrange to weigh them and immunize them at home.

- Take along a friend when you go to the clinic if you can. If not, a receptionist may be free to assist.
- Prams are often forbidden inside the clinic, but you can ask. Once it is appreciated what your problem is, you may find that an exception can be made.
- If you are organized, you may like a tip from TAMBA that several mothers find helpful: weigh the babies fully clothed, then subtract the weight of identical clothes you have put in the changing bag just for this purpose.

· *Coping at Home in the First Year* ·

The only point of having baby equipment is to make life safer for your babies and easier for yourself. You can go overboard on such things and even if your house is ample in size you could soon find yourself squeezed out by all the 'essentials' you have acquired without getting much benefit from them. So how best to use what is available?

Play-pens

You can do very well without a play-pen, but many mothers find them useful for safety if nothing else. Your babies can play in one reasonably unmolested if you have a jealous toddler; you can pop your babies in the play-pen when you answer the door or go to the loo; they are also handy in the garden. A play-pen could also be a good place for a daytime nap.

A second-hand play-pen is usually fine, but good solid construction is essential since two babies give it twice as much of a battering. It is tempting to use it a lot if you have multiples, as many mothers admit, but try not to overdo it. Even with loads of playthings, babies don't benefit from many hours in a play-pen because they miss out on personal attention and on interacting with the wider world. Besides, if you keep dumping them in the play-pen they may begin to hate it.

Highchairs

You will need highchairs some time in the first year, usually between five and eight months, when your twins sit up to eat. Always use a proper harness as well. Supervise your babies even when they are eating finger-food unaided: they may choke on a rusk. They also tend to pinch each other's food! Folding highchairs obviously save space.

Now that highchairs are widely available in family restaurants, you usually need no special arrangements when eating out, but if you need three or more highchairs, it is wise to ring first and request them.

There is an ingenious cloth harness called a Tam-Sit that, with the help of a cushion, turns most ordinary dining chairs into a safe seat for a baby. This is useful when travelling.

Baby-bouncers, baby-gyms etc.

These are seats that hang from a frame or doorway and your baby bounces up and down in it. The fun tends to last only a few minutes per session, so most mothers of twins cannot be bothered with them. However, the fun lasts much longer if you have two baby bouncers, and two door frames close together, so that the babies can see each other.

Baby-walkers

These little seats on wheels can be great fun, once a baby can sit up well. They also make a good place to put a baby when you answer the door, for example, but they have drawbacks:

- They are dangerous if they tip up and if used near the top of the stairs.

- Anyone not inside the baby walker gets his hands and feet run over. If you have twins, you will need two walkers, or else none. When you have two or three baby-walkers around, it can seem like the dodgems at a fair.

- Excessive use may be damaging and could even delay learning to walk.

All in all, you probably won't want to buy any baby-walkers, but it may be useful to borrow a couple from friends and use them only for short periods of time.

Keeping an eye on your babies

Babies are mobile fairly early on, usually crawling from about seven or eight months and standing at eight to ten months. Even before this they can get into serious trouble, however. Anything small tends to be investigated by mouth, so watch out for things such as beads, buttons, small batteries (especially harmful if swallowed) and Lego belonging to an older sibling.

As soon as your babies are a couple of months old, look out for potential dangers. Try to see your home from their point of view and remove or alter hazardous features. You can get lots of tips and advice from RoSPA (Royal Society for the Prevention of Accidents) and CAPT (Child Accident Prevention Trust) (see Resources, page 343).

However hard you try, a totally childproof home does not exist (and it would probably be very dull if it did). There is no substitute for watching over your twins constantly. Bathtime is particularly dangerous and you should never leave one or more babies alone in any bath. They can drown in less than 2.5 cm (an inch) of water: babies have been known to perish in the fluid at the bottom of a nappy bucket. As for your own ablutions, you may have to take the twins with you to the bathroom.

Safety gates are almost essential and you may need them for a long time. The fixed type, screwed into the wall, is more bother but much sturdier and especially useful at the top of the stairs. You need a gate at the bottom of the stairs too.

It can be handy to have a movable gate used across doorways as needed, for instance to keep your babies out of the kitchen. Even here you may prefer a fixed gate: whatever you use has to withstand a lot of punishment because two or more infants can pull down a gate more easily than a singleton of the same age.

· *Playing* ·

Young babies need to play with things, even if they only look at them. Details of the various possibilities – mobiles, cot toys, soft balls, mirrors, cloth books, music boxes, etc. – are outside the scope of this book, however. The question is, how many of what should you buy? You don't have to duplicate everything. You may want two of some things, like rattles, but even these needn't be identical. You need only one of some bigger items. It really depends on you, your budget and the space available.

Buying toys can be very expensive, which is where toy libraries come in. Remember also that many playthings – egg cartons, cotton reels, etc. – are free and can be a lot of fun.

Talking and eye contact are the best games of all, especially for multiples, and cost only time. Babies enjoy (and learn from) being smiled at, tickled, held, stroked, sung to, talked to and read to, long before they can speak. This sort of entertainment comes naturally to many mothers, who play spontaneously with babies, but others may be self-conscious and find it difficult.

It probably doesn't matter whether you make a fool of yourself in front of your babies or read to them from *The Times*, as one mother did. Your attention is all-important, particularly when provided on an individual basis for each baby, even if only for a few minutes at a time. If you can't manage this, play with your babies together, but try to establish eye contact with each.

· *Identity* ·

Most mothers have only one baby at a time and it is entirely normal to want to cherish and even brag about your babies' 'twin-ness'. You can still revel in this, and in your status as a parent of twins, while helping your babies achieve their own unique potential. All the evidence is that multiples grow up to function best when they are treated as individuals in their own right   and that means right from the beginning.

Time is your greatest enemy. It is expedient to lump twins or triplets together, to talk to them at the same time and to treat them generally as one unit. A child-minder once told me that caring for eight-month-old twins was no different from looking after one baby. While I was glad she felt that competent, it made me think about looking around for some other arrangement.

You can help your babies in many ways. First, encourage people to use their names. Nobody should be allowed to call them 'Twins' when talking to them. Referring to them as 'the babies' or 'the girls/boys' is a bit better, but ideally their own names should be used from the start.

This is not always as straightforward as it might seem. The French psychologist René Zazzo found that 10 per cent of parents couldn't recall which baby had originally been given which name! Also, even when you know perfectly well who is who, you can still say the wrong name when you are in a hurry (just as one occasionally slips up and uses a son's name when addressing one's husband).

Using the right names is a good start but fostering individuality ultimately depends on giving individual attention. Whenever you can, talk to each baby separately rather than addressing them collectively. This is an effort and you will inevitably end up saying such things as 'Look, a tree' rather more times than the average parent. It is worth it, however.

Frequent separate outings are a good idea all round. They will help you relate to each baby and will help them get individual attention. Many twins are never out of each other's sight and this will begin to tell later on: some will find it very traumatic if they have to endure a short separation, perhaps because one of them goes into hospital, for example.

Outings needn't always be ambitious. At this age, even going down to the corner shop, perhaps in a borrowed single buggy, can be exciting. If you have never had the pleasure of a singleton's company, it could be something of a novelty for you too.

Any helpers or child-carers you have should make it easier for you to arrange individual outings, as long as you have explained that these are important. Unfortunately, this does not always work out. Grandparents, for instance, may fail to see the point, or there may be an older sibling who is in her own way very needy of time and attention.

It can seem very hard at times to give both (or all) your offspring the right amount of attention. What is the right amount, anyway? If we're honest, most of us sometimes allot our time unequally, perhaps because one baby is easier, healthier or just more attractive. One baby may also get more attention because he's the one who constantly clamours for it.

At some point in the first year, you will probably notice how different your twins are in personality, even if they are officially identical. Dissimilarities are sometimes noticeable from very early on.

Both had an untraumatic birth – I had a caesarean without going into labour – and both weighed exactly the same. Alistair was the placid one from the first day, but Gareth would startle very easily, especially if anyone brushed against his hospital cot and made it swing. It only swung by a few degrees but he seemed to hate it and his limbs would jerk out. Alistair was in a type of cot that didn't move at all, so I swapped them round. Gareth settled, and the swinging cot never bothered Alistair at all.

It is all too easy for parents of twins to focus on differences and magnify them. We want our children to be individuals and perhaps it is easier to relate to them once we establish who is 'the quiet one', 'the smiley one', 'the greedy one', or whatever. Beware of labelling! Such distinctions may be real enough at the time, but often they are merely temporary. As soon as you have decided who the naughty one is and who the good one is, your youngsters may reverse roles in the next few weeks, just to keep you on your toes. Nobody really knows why this 'see-sawing' happens, but it is a well-known occurrence with multiples.

Most parents would agree that, regardless of their personal preferences, it is important to be fair as far as possible. In fact the great majority of parents seem to do very well in this respect. If you suspect that you are not, stop and analyse what you are doing and how you are spending your time. The chances are that you are doing a lot better than you imagine, but if you are worried you can always talk this over with someone at TAMBA Twinline (see page 343).

· *Clothes* ·

You will obviously want baby clothes that are easy to care for: not only machine-washable but also non-iron and preferably able to go in the tumble-drier. Your babies will soon grow and there are limits as to how much you can dry on radiators.

You may have noticed some babies wearing 'pram shoes'. These are not a good idea, especially for multiples. One twin's pram shoes could inflict damage on his sibling and, besides, you won't have time for such things. Shoes are superfluous until your babies begin to walk properly out of doors. Until then, padded slip-on elasticated footwear (such as 'Padders') with non-slip soles are all they need. When they do get their first shoes, have them measured properly and choose, if you possibly can, a time-saving style with a Velcro closure rather than buckles or laces.

Should you dress your babies alike or differently? Twins or more look very cute dressed identically and fit in with most people's concept of 'twin-ness'. In the very early days, it doesn't much matter how you dress them as long as you (and anyone else looking after them) can distinguish them easily. This is important, not just on safety grounds (twins have been known to end up with a double dose of antibiotics because their child-minders could not tell them apart) but also for relating to them as individuals on a daily basis.

Soon, though, it does matter very much how they are dressed. Twins as young as nine months will often notice what they are wearing: they have been known to get upset even at this tender age if they are suddenly dressed differently. Besides, the rest of the world needs to learn to distinguish between them, and clothes are a good start.

Perhaps it would be better for other people to learn to tell your babies apart on other grounds, such as facial features, personality, height or voice, for instance, but in practice it is better if you make it easier for them. Hairstyles don't help at this age: infants don't have enough hair!

The same outfits in different colours are an attractive way to dress multiples, but sticking too rigidly to colour codes can store up trouble for later on. Some twins may reject their school uniforms (or, as mine did, their PE bags in house colours) on the grounds that it is not 'their' colour.

Another method is to dress them in similar colours but differently styled clothes. This can look especially attractive on young triplets and boy–girl pairs, who may not otherwise look much like multiples.

Alternatively, you could forget about matching outfits altogether, which is obviously a lot easier because you can put them in whatever comes to hand in the morning. However, most mothers find it is quite a good idea for each baby to have his own clothes, except perhaps for boring items like vests.

You will inevitably be given sets of identical clothes for your babies, at least in the very early days. Nevertheless, you need not dress them the same: you can allocate, say, both turquoise sleepsuits to one baby and give the two yellow ones to his sister.

· *Weaning* ·

Your babies will be ready for solids at about four months old. This is only an approximate guide, because multiples are often small and may need solids later than singletons. One clue that a baby needs solids is when he reverts to night feeds a few weeks after you thought he'd given them up for good.

In general, it is best to try both or all your babies on solids at the same time, unless they are very different in health. Bear in mind, though, that one may take to solid food first.

The principles of starting solids are just the same as for a single baby, but the mess is greater. If you haven't had a baby before, you may be shocked by how much food ends up on the outside rather than the inside of your babies. This advice will help:

- Sit the babies in bouncing cradles or car seats to start with (or in a buggy if you are out), moving on to highchairs as they become better at sitting up.

- Don't use your sitting-room for meals if you can help it. The kitchen is ideal if you have the space. Spread newspapers out on the floor beneath the babies. You can use plastic sheeting, but it is tedious to wipe it every time; newspaper can be thrown away after each meal.

- Put on the answering machine if you have one. (Incidentally, a message with a background of crying babies is most effective in explaining why you cannot get to the phone at the moment. Using the same taped message when you are out could convince a potential burglar that you are in.)

- Use plastic bibs with a pelican-type trough. At the end of the meal you can just tip out the slop. These bibs don't last long; they crack with frequent use, so replace them as necessary.

- In warm weather, the babies can be stripped down to nappy and vest to avoid washing clothes more than necessary.

- Multiples tend to share germs, so, unless there are compelling medical reasons, use one spoon and one bowl for both (or all) babies. Feed a spoonful to each in turn, stopping only to fill up the spoon. You will find that once they get the hang of it, they sit up with their mouths permanently open like tiny birds and you will hardly be able to keep up with demand. Many mothers and any onlookers find this very cute.

- So that they still grasp the idea of cutlery, you can give your babies a spare plastic spoon each to hold, wave about, bash against the highchair, etc.

- Try to take it in your stride if they have different tastes. Unless there are definite allergies, they should still be offered the same foods (catering now for their preferences could be troublesome later). If you don't go to a lot of trouble to prepare tasty meals, you will be less upset when they reject them.

- Ice-cube trays are often suggested for freezing portions of home-prepared baby food, but empty yoghurt pots, cottage cheese containers, etc. are a better size with twins or more.

- Finger-foods come into their own from about six months and your babies may have fun trying to feed each other. This is also a time when they will want to try feeding themselves – a messy but essential experiment. The temptation with multiples is to spoon-feed them for as long as possible to minimize chaos and save time, but they must be allowed to learn, even if they use their yoghurt as finger-paint. You will have many more problems later if you don't let them play around with feeding themselves as soon as they are ready.

- If you are eating at the same time, which becomes possible once the babies get to finger-foods, try to set a good example. With luck, they might just copy you. As they get older, it becomes more important to take your meals with them.

- Training them to sit still for meals even without a high-chair is quite easy towards the end of the first year. Sit them on a blanket or sheet. Just remove the food if they get up. Later, they may even eat their sandwiches at picnics without crawling away mid-meal.

- In the early days, you will be finishing off each session of solids with a bottle (or breast), but try to get your babies on to cups or drinkers when you can. Most babies go through a stage at about six months when they really take to a beaker, which is much better for them: drinks from bottles are more likely to damage developing teeth.

- Sometimes one baby will give up the breast or bottle first and the other follows within a few weeks. Meanwhile, you can enjoy the closeness of feeding just one.

· *Sleep* ·

Soon after the age of six months, babies acquire the ability to stay awake deliberately (and apparently indefinitely) even when they, and you, are worn out. They can of course also be kept awake by discomfort, hunger, illness or teething, causes which you may need to consider and rule out.

In many ways, sleepless twins differ little from sleepless singletons, but their impact is greater because caring for their day-to-day needs is more demanding. If your babies do not sleep at the same time, their individual habits need not be particularly problematic for you to suffer.

It may be hard to enjoy your twins if they are responsible for waking you night after night. Youngsters who sleep poorly can also be a distinct drain on relationships within the rest of the family, perhaps especially if you and your partner have agreed between you that you must bear the brunt of the night-time duties so that he can get enough sleep to function at the office.

It is often said that nobody ever died from lack of sleep, but psychologists in industry are beginning to question this old saw. In everyday life, lack of sleep can lead to constant tiredness and symptoms of depression, and can seriously impair one's effectiveness at home or at work.

Patterns of sleeplessness vary from baby to baby. Some youngsters have trouble getting off to sleep, while others wake repeatedly for no apparent reason. Some babies start waking again for a night feed, especially around the age of four or five months, but this is often a sign that they need more food, or need to start solids. It is hunger and has nothing to do with most babies' sleeping problems. Some babies may continue to sleep erratically or only for short periods because that is what they did in the early days and weeks. In other cases it may be because they have always nodded off at the breast or on the bottle before being put into their cots.

However in most babies the cause of sleeplessness is not at all obvious.

The question is, what to do about it? Many parents find it comforting to know that they are not alone, that their babies' poor sleeping habits are not their fault, that their parenting is not inadequate, and that things will improve in time. Indeed they will, but for the time being this is not always enough.

Many things have helped parents of under-ones avert serious sleep problems, such as:

- a room which is comfortable, being neither too cold nor too warm
- a regular bedtime
- a pleasant and predictable bedtime routine
- going in to check a crying baby but not picking him up
- night attire which is comfortable, without tight sleeves, constricting wristbands, and so on
- night-lights or, paradoxically, dark curtains/curtain lining
- dummies
- keeping any night-feeds and nappy changes as brief and business-like as possible
- learning to relax yourself
- snatching a siesta whenever you can.

Should your babies sleep in the same room? Some multiples seem to disturb each other, but others may gain satisfaction from being in the same room. There are no fixed rules, and you will soon know what kind of individuals your babies are.

If their sleeplessness causes trouble, it will certainly help to

- talk over your difficulties with your health visitor
- contact Twinline or CRY-SIS (see pages 343 and 344)
- read the TAMBA leaflet on sleeping problems in multiples (which also covers toddlers and older children).

There are several tried and tested approaches for established sleeping problems. One, sometimes called the checking method, is to keep checking but not picking up a crying baby. Go to your child when he cries and let him know you are nearby. Instead of lifting him, however, simply tuck him in or pat him, then say goodnight and leave. He may wail again (if he has stopped at all), but do not return to him for three to five minutes. Use a watch to time yourself as it will seem endless. Gradually lengthen the time interval between checks. This firm approach is also called the controlled crying method and is often recommended by health visitors and many other childcare experts. It may sound cruel, but you are not being unkind if you have already established there is nothing physically wrong. Many parents are delighted by how well it works, and it sometimes does the trick within a week or so. Others need longer. It is important to be consistent and confident, and of course to get the support of your partner too.

Withholding night-time drinks may help. Many young children who wake in the night are offered a drink to settle them, and this can perpetuate their wakefulness. If you gradually withdraw (usually by diluting with water) the night-time drinks, they may become too unexciting to bother with, and there is therefore less of an incentive to clamour for one. Water is also healthier for emerging teeth: recent reports show that even pure fruit juices can rot a youngster's teeth.

If your babies seem to wake each other, or perhaps one consistently wakes his twin, it may be a good idea to separate them at night, at least temporarily, if you can.

You will almost certainly succeed with one of these methods, or one of the other ideas from TAMBA. If not, some parents start considering giving one or both babies a sedative at bedtime. Most of these sedatives (for example Phenergan, Vallergan) have been around for many years, and in my experience as a GP are generally safe when used correctly.

However they should be prescribed by your doctor and used only for short periods of time. They do not always work but, in conjunction with behavioural methods, they can be effective when used for a week or so to break the pattern of sleeplessness or night-waking.

I am not suggesting that you sedate a baby on a long-term basis, or purely for your convenience. Equally, you should not have to feel guilty at having to ask your GP to consider prescribing a sedative. Make sure you tell your doctor how bad things are getting.

· *When They are ill* ·

Twins don't necessarily get ill simultaneously, but they sometimes do. When one or other is unwell, keeping both of them happy becomes a juggling act, especially if you have to carry the sick one around most of the time. Under these circumstances the well one may become particularly demanding. On the other hand, many mothers find that, thankfully, the opposite happens: the healthy one is content to make do with very little from you while his twin is ill.

With triplets or more, you are likely to feel very stretched during even minor illnesses. Episodes like this, says one mother of triplets, were the lowest points of their first year. Any help with any one of the babies is more than welcome. Now is the time to take up any offers you may have been rash enough to decline when all was well.

You will find that a fractious youngster is much easier to handle once any fever is controlled, so do give him paracetamol syrup or whatever your doctor has recommended for fever. Make sure he gets enough fluid to drink – you may have to tempt him often – and don't overwrap a sick baby.

Unless they are very ill, many sick babies can still go out in a pram or buggy, even if grandparents are horrified by this modern practice. Most babies appreciate a change of scene. If you really are confined to the house or flat, use different rooms at various times of the day if you can.

Don't worry about one ill baby infecting the other: there is nothing much you can do about it. All the same, each should have his own medicines. Babies shouldn't share prescriptions, only paracetamol and over-the-counter medicines.

Nor should your twins share medical records or a child health book. Treat each one as completely separate; even identicals don't always have the same allergies, for instance.

If one of your babies has to go into hospital, you must decide whether to take the other one too. The usual answer is no, unless you are breast-feeding or, perhaps as a single parent, have no option.

Hospitals nowadays are used to mothers staying the night with their baby. In fact, you may be relied on to provide much of the care. This will do a lot for your sick baby, though it is likely to exhaust you further. A grandparent who can stay and give you a hand when you get home is a great help.

· *Other Stresses* ·

The first year can be quite a strain all round. Your partner will have had to pitch in a lot, helping to care for the babies, doing domestic chores, giving you support, and carrying on with his own work, perhaps on little sleep. Meanwhile, older siblings' lives may have been turned upside down (a topic covered in Chapter 8).

Normal family activities may seem to have been abandoned, or exchanged for a never-ending round of chores. If you have help at home, you may have more time for each other and the children, but at the expense of less privacy.

Parents of triplets or more can have a particularly hard

time. The National Study of Triplets and Higher Order Births confirms that many triplet mothers have health problems in the first year, as do some of their partners. Many parents have found their relationship strengthened, but for some couples caring for multiples has the opposite effect and marital discord, even separation, is not unknown.

More help in the first year would no doubt make things easier, but there may be few offers. How many friends, for instance, are willing to take on two or more babies for a morning? This in turn has an isolating effect on a mother, who may feel her life is now totally out of control. Just getting out of the house seems an achievement in the early months, yet for many mothers that is not enough. Compared with her previous life, the rare outings she can now manage may appear very dull. And wherever she goes, she is a 'mother of twins', rather than herself. Going back to work at this stage may seem crazy, but for some mothers it becomes essential.

· *Making Life Easier* ·

Many mothers of twins later regret having spent so much of their time and energy on drudgery and chores in their babies' first year instead of being with them and enjoying family life. If they could have the time again, these women would do it differently. You can make it easier on yourself by re-examining your priorities in this crucially important year and by realizing now, before it is too late, that time is precious.

1   Get into a routine you can live with. The sooner your babies' habits are synchronized and simplified, the better. For instance, you still don't have to give them all daily baths: they don't get that dirty at this age. When you think about it, very little ironing is essential, either (it is also dangerous with babies around).

2   Get help if you can. Perhaps a friend's *au pair*, or a neighbour's teenaged daughter, could spare a few hours a week. She could bath the babies, do the shopping or perhaps give an older sibling his own outing. She could also make a big contribution by looking after one of your babies for an hour or two

3   If you are back at work, make sure your child-carer contributes to the domestic chores. If they go to a child-minder, can you enlist some other help with housework or washing? Note that a child-minder for two babies can work out expensive; you may be better off with someone who comes to your house. It is normal for nannies to do the children's washing and keep their rooms clean, but could she also wash the kitchen floor? Negotiate at the outset. Unqualified nannies are often more flexible on this, and not necessarily less experienced than qualified ones.

4   Make a point of playing with your babies and giving them attention. Go out regularly, for instance to toddler groups, no matter how hard it seems at the time. Once you get there you will all benefit from socializing. Many mothers comment that a daily outing keeps them relatively sane.

5   Ignore comments that are plainly unhelpful and advice which doesn't apply to multiples. If you are a new parent, there will be plenty of them. You can acknowledge useless but well-meant suggestions with a non-committal 'I'll think about it.'

6   Banish guilt. If you've got this far and taken some of the ideas on board, you are probably doing well. There will be good days and less good days, but there is no need to punish yourself when you don't get things quite right. You can only do so much.

7   If you can afford it, consider taking a family holiday soon. Your twins probably aren't mobile yet and may be happy sitting in a pushchair for a while. Also, because they are under two years old, you may be able to enjoy some reasonably priced deals, but you'll probably have most fun if you try not to be too ambitious.

8   Make some time for yourself and your partner. However remote the future seems now, your children will eventually grow up and then where will you be?

· *The Light at the End of the Tunnel* ·

Most available research – and advice – on rearing twins concentrates on the hardships and difficulties of having more than one child at a time. There is no doubt this first year is a challenge, which makes it all the more necessary to give some thought to the joys of multiples – and there are plenty of those, believe me.

> Whenever I felt low in the first few months, I'd bundle my babies into their huge pram, which was the size of a skip, and head for the streets where I'd be bound to get gasps of admiration from total strangers.

> I'd come home from work and they'd cling to me like limpets, one on each of my legs. It certainly makes you feel wanted.

> After bathtime, they'd clamber all over me with their little pink bodies, still wet and glistening from the bath, and smelling fantastic. I'll never forget that baby smell.

The following list incorporates some personal views from parents as well as findings from research carried out by Dr Herbert Collier of Phoenix, Arizona, who, unusually, decided to focus a project on the pleasures of having twins.

- Twins (and more) are often amazingly cute-looking and stay that way much longer than most singletons. This is one reason why they attract so much attention, which many parents enjoy.

- It is fun to observe their individual personalities develop, at least twice as fascinating as with a singleton.

- Watching them interact is brilliant. Even at this tender age, they may smile and gurgle at each other and appear to have a tacit understanding.

- Soon you may also notice a special bond developing between the twins. Young twins sometimes learn to share things such as drinks, biscuits and toys quite spontaneously (however, don't bank on it).

- Even when they are not particularly close, twins have someone else to share life's joys and problems with and are a comfort to each other.

- Many parents of multiples say that, however shocked they were when they received the news, they somehow feel special, lucky or blessed.

- Fathers of twins often benefit from being far more involved in the day-to-day care of the children than they would have been with a singleton.

- You get double the joy, love, and cuddles (often from both at the same time).

- You do have to refocus your life, but this is often all to the good and can be an enriching experience which brings new friends and a new emphasis. Your career may even develop in a new direction.

- Once they get to the end of the first year, many mothers feel an intense sense of achievement. If you can manage twins, you can manage almost anything.

Chapter Seven

TODDLERS, OR THE TERRIBLE TWOS

Toddlerhood takes in the time between one and three years, or roughly the interval between learning to walk and starting playgroup or nursery. It is a time of emerging independence, increasing negativity, unbounded curiosity and learning new skills (for you as well as your babies).

Major toddler pastimes are finding out about the world, doing things for themselves and of course pushing you to the limit (just to establish what that is). What happens when one pulls the cat's tail, climbs the curtains or opens that fascinating door on the washing-machine?

From a practical point of view, the main difference between having one toddler and having two or more is that your attention is divided, which makes it more difficult to keep them occupied and out of trouble, especially when you are tired. With multiples, safety is a major issue and fighting is often another. There is more about fighting in Chapter 9, which deals with behaviour and language, while toddler topics are covered here.

· *Safety* ·

As you are watching over or playing with one toddler, you constantly have to bear in mind the other one (whoever said that there's safety in numbers wasn't a parent). Mothers of twins report a high incidence of injuries and accidents. In a survey for TAMBA, parents reported using more safety equipment with twins under five than when their older siblings were the same age. One particular danger highlighted was that rushing to the aid of one injured youngster often put the other twin at risk of injury.

Clearly, two or more can do more mischief. They egg each other on and they are physically capable of more: one small child cannot climb out of a play-pen, but she can if her brother lets her use his back as a step. Similarly, even settees and bookcases can be upturned by two determined toddlers.

> My two would use the banisters as a kind of game. Eloise climbed on the outside and Hilary on the inside, laughing and poking at each other between the bars until, inevitably, Eloise would either fall or be pushed off.

One toddler can jam the other one's fingers in a drawer and keep it painfully shut by leaning against it, or force the other's face down on to something as innocent as a piece of Duplo, necessitating a trip to Casualty for stitches (it has been known).

You are unlikely to get through toddlerhood totally without mishap, but you can reduce the risk of serious injuries by appreciating potential dangers and anticipating accidents. Anyone – their father, grandparent, child-minder, baby-sitter, etc. – who looks after the children also needs to be aware of hazards. Some mothers of twins point out that leaving Dad in charge often does not give the anticipated respite since fathers may be oblivious of many dangers.

Cupboard catches and latches are almost essential. They will stop or at least delay a toddler from getting at the contents, though they may not prevent one of your twins getting his fingers crushed in the door by his brother or sister. Don't rely totally on catches: all chemicals should be placed well out of reach, and medicines too. If some pills go missing, you may not even be able to tell the hospital which of your twins ate them.

A bolt high up on the inside of the front door will prevent your toddlers from running out into the street, but remove bolts and keys from bathroom and toilet doors, or fit a bolt high up where only you can reach it. Glass doors are an obvious hazard, so use safety glass, safety film and perhaps stickers. Consider putting removable bars on upstairs windows, especially in the children's bedroom.

Stair-gates will be very useful for a little while longer and you will soon be adept at climbing over them. Kitchens, with their knives, flexes and cookers, pose particular problems. A stair-gate across the kitchen door helps keep your twins safe while you cook.

Heaters must be protected by fire-guards. Avoid wall heaters and electric or open fires altogether if you can. Irons are best kept well out of the way: even a cooling iron can burn. Also, make sure your domestic hot water supply is not boiling hot; turn the thermostat down if necessary.

Twins often enjoy bathing together at this age and it is easier for you, but bathtime can be dangerous. Don't turn your back, even for two seconds, and never answer the phone or doorbell while they are in the bathroom. As a general guide, a child under the age of six is not safe on his own in the bath and, if unsupervised, even a seven-year-old is not safe in the bath with his twin. Friends with singletons may hardly believe this, but it's true.

For the sake of your nerves as much as anything else, put valuables and fragile belongings on a high shelf or in another room. It may save you having to say 'No' a hundred times a day.

I knew I had to remove all my favourite ornaments, like the china cats, but hadn't reckoned on the lamps. When I realized how fascinating my two found table lamps were, I removed them from the sitting room for about three years in all.

Thinking ahead saves you trouble. Keep your toddlers' fingernails short. Avoid toys like hammer pegs: twins are peculiarly prone to hammering each other's heads instead of the pegs. Toys with string or rope can also be dangerous: one may tie it around his brother's neck (or any other part of his anatomy) and pull for all he's worth. If you have an older child, keep an eye out for his toys. Quite apart from the fact that the twins could upset him by destroying them, they could prove lethal in younger hands.

Start keeping cot sides down from about eighteen months, so that when the children begin to climb out they will have less far to fall. It is sometimes during holidays that they develop in leaps and bounds. For obvious reasons, avoid bunk-beds until they are much older.

Don't forget that while you are keeping one toddler out of trouble, the other one could quietly wander off and get up to something else. I cannot emphasize enough how dangerous the world is with more than one toddler and it is impossible to list all the potential dangers. There is no such thing as a child-proof room: with two or more, as you soon discover, even a padded cell could be dangerous. Unless your toddlers are exceptionally placid, it is best not to let them out of your sight at this age. Supervise them, if only from a distance, while they explore. This will obviously affect your ability to give your children individual attention, but you just cannot do it all, and safety has to come first.

· *Individuality and Independence* ·

It is tempting to use collective nouns for your children (for example, twins, boys, gang, mob, twiglets, dynamic duo, awesome foursome) but this should be kept to a minimum, for their sakes. According to some experts, calling them 'Twins' is politically incorrect, but (as with all such matters) one can take this too far. It can be expedient to *refer* to them as 'the twins' or 'the triplets', although you should avoid *calling* them by these names when talking to them. Try your best to use their individual names, even if it is only to say, 'Anthony, leave that alone.'

At this age, giving individual attention when you can and addressing each child separately are all-important to their development in general and their language and behaviour in particular. Give each child time to talk to you, perhaps at bathtime or bedtime. Each needs to have his say in private sometimes.

Bedtime stories are a good way of winding down active toddlers and getting them in the mood for sleep, but one story or two? If you start reading to one while the other plays on the floor, you will soon find yourselves disturbed and interrupted. The ideal is to read to each child individually, with the other one in another room, perhaps getting a story from your partner, but few twins and even fewer triplets have this luxury. However, you may be able to do this at weekends, and during the week the children can share one story. Reading to them, whether separately or together, is a precious time for many parents.

Separate outings every so often are helpful, perhaps even separate overnight stays at a grandparent's house (especially since many grandparents find more than one toddler at a time too much to handle). It's best to stay flexible on this point and let it evolve naturally. Attempts to separate young twins for more than an hour or two can backfire, as some mothers discover. If each child thinks of a weekend with Grandma as a punishment, because they didn't want to be separated, this does nobody a favour.

· *Clothes* ·

For items such as underwear it won't matter, but on the whole your toddlers will prefer to have their own clothes, especially if you have a girl–boy pair. Dressing them differently, as suggested in the previous chapter, helps them to develop as individuals and the children will soon enjoy dressing and choosing their own clothes. It is also an important aid to safety. Toddlers should at the very least wear different outdoor clothes and wellingtons. A child who ventures out on to a busy road may well ignore an adult who calls him back by the wrong name, not because he is obstinate (though he may be) but because it isn't him who's being called.

Admittedly, there may be the odd occasion when it is useful for the children to be dressed similarly. One mother who lost one of her identical girls on a beach found her easily by explaining to strangers that she'd lost a child who looked 'just like this one'.

Nevertheless, they need not wear the same colours. When my two boys ran off in opposite directions in a shopping centre, I asked a passer-by to get 'the red one' while I ran after his brother, who was dressed in blue.

Dressing

It is one thing to get toddlers' clothes out and quite another to get them on. The worst ten minutes (or maybe hour) of your day is likely to be getting them ready in the morning. When they are very young, you have to dress them yourself, but it is not easy running after two or more toddlers who have so much more energy than you. Try to make dressing fun to encourage their co-operation:

- keep clothing simple
- be organized (getting clothes out the night before is a help)
- distract them while you dress them
- instead of rushing after them, try to get them to come to you.

It is expedient to keep dressing them yourself, just as it is to continue spoon-feeding them, but sometime after their second birthday your children will need to start putting on a few clothes themselves. Some mothers, especially if they have to get out of the house on time for work or to take an older child to school, find this stage absolutely maddening with twins, both of whom are determined to dress themselves, despite their complete incompetence at it. You just have to let them learn when they are ready, if necessary getting up earlier in the morning to do so. This stage lasts a long time with some children, but it passes eventually, and you will benefit in the end.

· *Fair but Different* ·

Life is not fair, but this is a hard lesson to learn, especially in early childhood. At this age, expectations of fairness are particularly high. If one twin gets a present or treat, or receives something which is in some way 'better', it is often seen by the other twin as a punishment.

Once they realize the extent to which jealousy and competition can exist between their children, parents try very hard to be fair. But inevitably there will be occasions when they are treated unequally, for instance parties, Cub Scouts, etc. In the longer run, it may be preferable for children not to be treated fairly, but this is very difficult to do and at this age it is better to be even-handed.

Generally, the younger the child, the more helpful it is for them to have presents which are roughly similar in concept or size, but presents needn't be identical. Although identical gifts are often acceptable, they can disappoint: if twins habitually receive the same birthday presents, once one child has opened his, the surprise is spoilt for his twin. (To some extent you can get round this by sitting the children back to back when they open their presents.)

For substantial presents, like a tricycle, the obvious choice would be the same but in different colours. Some toys, such as a Wendy house, can be shared between them, but obviously only one child at a time can use a bicycle or wheelbarrow so these are best duplicated. Besides, ownership is important to youngsters. If they do get one present between them – and this should be the exception, not the rule – you could also give them a tiny additional present each.

People can be amazingly unthinking and, as a parent, you may need to encourage everyone to give your twins or triplets individual presents. Birthday cards which read 'Happy Birthday, Twins' should also be banned. People buy them because they exist, but imagine how it must feel to have to share a card with someone else.

To set an example, you have to do your bit when giving other children presents. If they are going to a party, each of your twins should take a present for the birthday child. This needn't be expensive, but it may require a little imagination on your part.

Fair is not the same as equal; if you have one child with special needs, you know that already. It is better to give a child something she wants or that is appropriate for her. Adults sometimes fall into the trap of thinking they have to spend the same on each child. One aunt was convinced it was only fair to pay a certain amount for gifts for her twin nieces, aged four. One Christmas this entailed her giving two presents wrapped up together to Sarah and only one, albeit larger and more valuable, to Frances. Neither girl could comprehend this, however; Frances was very upset, while Sarah gloated.

There will be occasions when you have to assume that they both want roughly the same thing. For example if one child asks for a snack or a drink, it is sensible to offer one to his twin too, if only to save you getting up two minutes later.

Should you buy both twins clothes or shoes at the same time? You could spend a lot more if you do, so it is better to buy only for the one who actually needs new clothes. The other one may feel a bit left out, but in time he will learn to accept it as normal. An ice-cream for the one who has not got a new winter coat is unnecessary and may make things worse. If hand-me-downs are available, try to alternate who gets new and who gets second-hand – easier said than done if you have a boy–girl pair and, say, an older girl.

Like spouses, parents sometimes buy presents when they feel guilty, but this is never very satisfactory. On the whole, it is more important to be fair with time and attention than with money. Even this can be difficult, however. Within a mixed-sex pair, for instance, the girl may have a longer attention span and seem to need to be read to more. Differences will be more obvious if you have one child with special needs.

In time you will notice many other differences between your twins. One may be placid, the other demanding or adventurous. One may smile and laugh a lot, while her twin is grumpy. As in the first year, labelling has its dangers throughout your twins' childhood. It is one thing to encourage differences – and later you may want to make use of these in, for instance, the choice of a musical instrument to learn or a sport to play – but it is quite another to polarize the children. Like prophecies, exaggerations occasionally become self-fulfilling. More often, though, labels don't last.

> For several weeks, Amanda was a sweet-natured toddler and butter wouldn't melt in her mouth. Zoe, meanwhile, would grizzle and grump. But, lo and behold, for no reason at all they suddenly swapped and now Amanda behaved as if she had the devil in her.

Twins, especially if identical, may change over, seemingly just to fool you. This phenomenon, also mentioned in the previous chapter, can be very marked in toddlerhood, but it is seen in twins throughout childhood and probably has a lot to do with the division of labour and perception of roles within the twinship.

· *Tantrums* ·

You may think that if you are scrupulously fair, all will be well. Alas, toddlers don't operate like that. Tantrums are an inevitable part of growing up and most toddlers between the ages of two and three have at least one a week. They probably result from a child knowing exactly what he wants but failing to understand why he cannot have it there and then.

Children do grow out of them, but twins – especially boys – tend to go on having tantrums long after most singletons have given them up. You may find that one of your toddlers flies off the handle more readily than the other, or that they set each other off.

> I found that only Paul would start tantrumming, but if I got overheated in the process, David would go bananas too, perhaps from fear.

You can help prevent tantrums by:

- being consistent but firm
- giving your toddlers plenty of attention
- giving way on unimportant issues (this is not a bad principle whatever your children's age, even in the teen years)
- avoiding unnecessary temptations, such as the super market check-out with all the chocolates
- setting a good example yourself: chances are that with two or more young children you are doing a lot of shouting, if only to make yourself heard, but it pays to keep the emotional temperature down.

During a tantrum, shouting or smacking usually prolong the agony for all concerned. A hug can help calm a child, but he may just need to be left, as long as you keep an eye on him to make sure he's safe. Meanwhile, don't forget his twin: he may take the opportunity to wander off and cause some quiet mischief while you are dealing with his brother's outburst.

After the storm, carry on as if it hadn't happened. It shouldn't alter anything. If you weren't going to buy him a sweetie, don't get him one now. This is hard, especially if your toddlers have chosen to tantrum in unison in the supermarket, but they have to learn that blowing an emotional fuse is useless. (See Chapter 9 for more on bad behaviour in general.)

· *Potty-Training* ·

Many mothers dread this stage, but potty-training two or more toddlers doesn't usually turn out to be the awful experience some expect. It is, however, apt to be very messy, since it's hard to keep an eye on both at once. That is, assuming your twins are ready to come out of nappies simultaneously. They may not be and, even with identicals, there can be an interval of months between them. Children also vary in the order they develop: some have bladder control before bowel control and vice versa.

> They were both ready together when they were two and a half. Once they both did poos just as they'd got up from their potties and they both trod it into the carpet. Weeing was less of a problem, though both girls usually managed to store at least one settee's worth of wee in their bladders, to be released as soon as my back was turned.

If you've done it before, you know that the key to successful potty-training is not to rush it. Forcing the issue is counterproductive, so ignore bragging mothers, including yours if she claims you were clean by nine months (as Gladstone was said to be). Babies of this age are not sufficiently developed neurologically to control the muscles involved;

your mother was probably just 'catching' your poos in a potty.

Watch for signs that one of your toddlers is ready: he may start expressing a distaste for dirty nappies, or pull off his nappy when it is wet or dirty.

Other things being equal, start potty-training in warm weather soon after the children's second birthday. There are two main methods, but either way you need enough potties and eternal vigilance. Keep their clothing simple and easy to remove, or leave their bottoms bare altogether.

Either sit your children on their potties for ten minutes or so at a time (or however long the toddler is happy with). At this stage, youngsters know what toilets and potties are for, so just wait till they produce something or get bored. The bowels often empty about twenty minutes after breakfast, so this is a good time. Congratulate the one who produces a result, but don't go overboard in your praise. If you show too much appreciation your child may end up offering you 'gifts' of his stools!

Alternatively, take off your toddlers' nappies for an hour or two to begin with, then for longer and longer. Keep the potties handy but don't make either child sit on them unless you see signs of, for instance, jumping about, holding the crotch, wriggling or crouching down quietly in a corner. You will inevitably have many accidents, but one day success will come.

Don't worry or lose heart if only one toddler gets the idea. Often the other will want to emulate this achievement a few weeks later and, as some mothers have found, twins practically train each other. Just be patient. However, watch out for the toddler who empties his potty triumphantly over his twin's head.

You will soon reach the stage where you take potties with you when you go out. Dressing your children in terry pants for outings is useful, as are old towels in the seat of the buggy. Fortunately, most buggies wash quite easily under a garden hose.

Toddlers will of course still need nappies at night for a while, perhaps till the age of three or more. Throughout childhood, plastic mattress covers will save you time and effort. It is not just bowels and bladders you have to consider – there may be vomit or nosebleeds as well!

· *Playing* ·

Playing is something toddlers do instinctively, but some aspects of play are subtly (or not so subtly) different with multiples. For example, toys are more likely to be used as weapons. Though it can happen, a singleton is unlikely to poke himself in the eye with a pencil, for instance, and rocking-horses can squash little fingers. For this reason, many playthings suitable for your children's age should be regarded as hazardous with two or more. You will also need to supervise your children more closely when they play.

Unless they are very robust, toys get broken more easily with multiples, causing disappointment all round.

Multiples make more mess and you may decide to abandon experiments such as finger-painting. However, you could let them paint outside, or on a plastic table-cloth on the floor. One mother, realizing she had two young graffiti artists, allowed them to draw on one designated wall outside the downstairs toilet. 'This worked very well,' she reported, 'though they did bicker over how much wall they should each have, until I painted a vertical line down the middle.'

Outdoors, a swing can be downright dangerous. The seat of the moving swing can hit the other twin on the head and knock her unconscious. See-saws are often considered a brilliant idea for twins, but can cause injuries and thus rarely work out well. If you are considering getting outdoor toys, you are better off with a slide, trampoline, Wendy house or, best of all, a sandpit. This will exercise their imaginations yet consume hardly any of your energy.

There are positive aspects, especially when toddlers co-operate. They may take turns wheeling each other around in a play wheelbarrow (until, that is, one gets fed up and violently tips out his twin). Imaginative play tends to work very well with twins or more: there is no shortage of customers when playing restaurants, or of patients when playing hospitals.

You will find that playing or reading with them is enjoyable and also prevents arguments, which results in less stress for you, but it is hard, if not downright impossible, to play with one and not the other. One twin will want to muscle in on whatever the other one is doing and your attention will be divided. Obviously, the presence of a sensible older child or another adult is helpful, but most of us have to manage on our own as best we can.

A frequent problem with twins is fighting over toys. When they fight they tend to do it with the gloves off, without much awareness of the damage they inflict. Who owns what? Some toys may be 'sharing' ones, but what about the Duplo and other bricks? If each has his own, they either play separately or co-operate and get the bricks muddled up – and then squabble.

> When they do fight, I take that toy away and offer them something else, or preferably a choice of several toys, to interest them. At this age, memories are mercifully short!

It is a good idea for each child to have his own toys, although you'll naturally want to avoid unnecessary (and expensive) duplication. Owning things is probably a basic human instinct, while taking turns is less so. A child who has his own playthings and his own box or shelf to store them:

- may be more careful with them
- may learn (eventually) to put them away
- may fight less
- finds it easier to choose what he'd like as a present.

Of course, each can still share with his twin and this is delightful to watch when it happens, though it is not something you can rely on for a few years yet.

· *Getting Out and About* ·

You will still be using the buggy for most outings. A couple of toys in a bag are useful to keep your toddlers amused. Alternatively, take a small selection of reading matter: toddlers devour books, often literally.

It is tempting to keep twins in their buggy till the age of four or so, but they need to walk. The trouble is that it is often in different directions. So when they seem ready to get out and walk, let them, but take the buggy along, just in case they get tired or fed up.

Reins that double as pushchair harnesses give you flexibility. Leather reins tend to work better than fabric. Reins also give your children freedom, though they can get tangled up (more so, inevitably, with triplets).

The fact that twins use a buggy for longer may have an effect on road awareness, but most mothers seem to think it doesn't make much difference. In practice, you cannot trust any child under five to cross the road safely and he may be unreliable for years longer. There is evidence that real traffic awareness is pretty rudimentary until the age of eleven or so.

On car journeys, singing or listening to cassettes helps keep toddlers occupied and reasonably under control. According to research, nursery rhymes may even be a valuable aid to language development – if you can stand the repetition.

In the car, the main trouble with multiples at this stage is likely to be screaming, shouting or scratching each other, any of which could cause your own attention to wander. If this happens, just pull in and get them to stop.

> I was against smacking but had no qualms about giving a sharp tap if they were acting up. Screaming and howling while we're on the motorway is definitely too dangerous to allow.

Another difficulty is the buckle on the child seat. It depends a bit on the model of the seat, but some youngsters soon discover that they can undo the buckle. Again, this is something you need to act on swiftly as it can be extremely dangerous.

Getting toddlers into and out of the car can be a pain if you have to do it more than a couple of times a day, and sometimes they nod off in the car seat just when you need to get out. If you are picking up an older child from school, you could ask another parent to bring her out to your car for you when this happens.

Taxis may seem appealing – after all, you wouldn't have to keep your eyes on the road as well as on the children – but the absence of child seats often makes them impractical with twins or more. If you try to restrain two slithering toddlers single-handedly on a meandering road, you will see why.

Shopping trips will continue to require a lot of energy for a little while. Leaving one child with a friend makes things easier. If you use two supermarket trolleys, make sure your children are both harnessed in: they can easily fall out as they try to grab things off the shelves. Also, be careful not to injure your back; many mothers have back problems. For clothes shopping, using one of the many good mail-order firms could be the most satisfactory solution.

· *Leisure* ·

Yes, you will get a chance to go out and enjoy yourselves, though some outings may be more stressful than they might have been with only one youngster in tow. Even going to the park is demanding if toddlers decide to career off in different directions. An enclosed children's play area is obviously easier, although it still leaves you with the problem of pushing two in swings at the same time.

Dress your children simply for such outings, with wellingtons if wet, so that you don't mind if they get messy. After all, part of the fun of a rainy day is stamping about in puddles.

For safety's sake, it is inadvisable to go swimming with children this young unless another adult comes along to help in the water, as well as with changing before and after. Formal swimming lessons may also be out of the question, since some instructors insist on one adult per child. It may be better to wait till your children are a bit older, then enrol them in a class where a parent is not required to be in the water. Don't worry if this means your children cannot swim until, say, the age of six or seven. They may be a bit disadvantaged socially, but not on grounds of safety: a young child who can swim a little in a warm calm pool is no safer than a non-swimmer if he happens to fall into an icy canal or a choppy sea.

Theme parks and funfairs are especially hard to manage without adult help. Many mothers find outings like these so demanding that they are simply not worth the effort (or the expense). You may feel that your children aren't getting many treats, but these things will get easier as they get older, when they are also more able to appreciate them. Besides, however much fun they are made out to be, theme parks are not one of life's essentials. A varied and stimulating home environment, with plenty of adult attention, and opportunities to make friends locally are good enough. Make the most of the outings you do make: talk with your toddlers about what you've seen and done. Don't forget to make eye contact with the child you are having the conversation with.

· *Going Visiting* ·

Going to see friends can be exhausting for you if your twins overwhelm the host, especially one with only a single toddler. It can also be embarrassing if they break things while you are not looking. There may be tears all round. When visits turn out badly, you may conclude that it is just not worth the effort of going out to see friends. However, you can make it easier on yourself.

- Ask your friend to hide away the most fragile objects and her child's most prized possessions. Perhaps her child could agree beforehand on what toys (if any!) he is willing to share with your tribe.
- Break up the visit with a meal, a picnic or just a walk in the park. Being outdoors helps burn off energy.
- Meet somewhere neutral: the park or a soft-play area at the leisure centre, for instance.
- Attempt short visits rather than day-long marathons.
- Use these gatherings strictly for the children's benefit and give up trying to say much to your friend. You can always catch up with them on the phone some other time.
- Visit at times such as weekends, when you or your friend may have another adult around to keep an eye on the children.
- Take only one of your toddlers with you if possible. Better still, organize a morning's exchange with another

parent of twins of a similar age, so that you have one of her children and she has one of yours. Many mothers consider this to be an ideal solution to the problems of visiting and helping their children develop as individuals.

- If things aren't working out, you may have to give up visiting friends for a few weeks, but don't leave it so long that you turn into a recluse.

· *Having Friends Round* ·

Similarly, your children may overwhelm a visiting child, or refuse to share their toys. The twins may even spend the afternoon fighting with each other over the right to play with the visitor, with the result that she toddles off to amuse herself on her own.

If they are in a particularly wicked mood, your children may gang up against the guest, despite the fact that they were all best pals yesterday at toddler group. A rough and unequal struggle can result, especially when things start getting thrown about.

Speaking to other parents of twins shows that, unfortunately, such behaviour is not unusual. Some add that having friends over to play was a problem that persisted for years, well into their twins' schooldays. Here, parents of triplets can find themselves at a distinct advantage. One mother reports that her problems were invariably over if she invited one child in to play with her three girls.

If you have twins:

- Invite two children over to play.
- Try swapping one child for a couple of hours with another parent with twins.
- Have one little friend round while one of your toddlers goes to a grandparent, aunt, or to visit another friend.

- Play a game with one of your children while the other one plays with the visitor (not easy, but it can work).

You may find you have to give up having friends over for a while, until your children can cope with their jealousy and competition. If so, try not to worry unduly. Although it is stimulating for them to mix with other children, they are unlikely to make real friendships outside the family until they are at least three years old. By this time, they may be at playgroup or nursery, which will give them new and different opportunities to socialize.

· *Birthday Parties* ·

At last, one area where twins or triplets really do lead to economies of scale! In the early years, one party for both (or all) is plenty. Besides, friends and relatives are shared at this age. Even later on, sharing a birthday tends not to be a big issue for the kids, though some parents still worry about it.

However, they shouldn't have to share presents or cards, so discourage people from giving these jointly. If each twin has suggested his own guest-list, you could ask each guest to bring a present just for the child who invited him (this works only if each twin invites the same number of friends). Nor should children have to blow out the same candles on the cake. You could have two cakes, or two sets of candles on the cake. This works well for several years if you have a cake in the shape of a log, say, or a train (until there are too many candles). Most parents of multiples sing 'Happy Birthday' as many times as they have children.

Watch out for games which only one person can win, such as musical chairs. You may find one of the toddlers elated from his win, while his twin is either in the slough of despond or throwing a tantrum (not unusual at birthday parties anyway, even with singletons). You can try playing pass-the-parcel with two parcels, or opt for less competitive games. Try to avoid situations where one or more children who are 'out' are left to rampage around the house getting into mischief. Here another adult is a great help.

· *How to Get Through a Difficult Day* ·

Most toddlers not only get into everything but seem to do it all on much less sleep than before. Giving up one or both daytime naps is something you have to get used to around now. You can, for a while anyway, encourage them to nod off by wheeling them around the streets in their buggy at strategic times of the day, or going for a drive in the car. If your toddlers still sleep in the day, use this time for your-self, not for chores. If only one dozes at a time, make the most of it by spending a few uninterrupted moments with the other child. He will benefit and so may you. Many a wild child becomes delightfully manageable on his own.

How else can you cope with all your toddlers' energy, especially when your own get-up-and-go has got up and gone?

1   Minimize chores. Postpone or give up any non-essential housework and enlist your children's help to do some of the others. Your toddlers could be kept busy 'polishing' the banisters while you vacuum. Admittedly, every-thing takes longer with their 'help', but they may enjoy it, it will keep them occupied and you will at least get something done.

2   Try to get through one day at a time without conflict, even when you have to repeat yourself like a tape loop to keep your toddlers out of trouble. It is less inflamma-

tory to tell them off by calling them 'silly' rather than 'stupid'.

3   Keep toys reasonably tidy, so that they are not all out at once. Mess creates stress: also, something should be hidden away, in reserve. Fortunately, there is no need to be meticulously tidy – it is said to inhibit play and discovery!

4   Have one or two activities or big toys that use up energy, for instance trampolining or bouncing on an old mattress on the floor. Or just get a few giant cardboard boxes to play around with (but watch out for any sharp staples).

5   Have at least one outing a day. Toddler groups and one o'clock clubs are good ways of burning off excess energy and you might even get to sit down.

6   Use different rooms for a change. Your toddlers could scribble at the kitchen table for a while, then play with bricks in the bedroom, before blowing bubbles out in the garden or the bathroom. You could even picnic in your garden or in the shed if it is big enough.

7   Use television wisely. There are a few excellent programmes for the very young. However, sitting glued to the set for too long can make children unbearably over-active later.

8   When they get restless, you can put on some music and dance together. A few crisps and a couple of drinks make it into an impromptu party.

9   Try not to let your children get overtired. If they are whiny and worn out but won't nap, you could sit and read to them together. Enjoying books quietly doesn't

take much energy on anyone's part and helps develop language skills.

10 Toddlers cannot usually go straight to sleep when they've been jumping about just before bedtime. Twins especially tend to overexcite each other, so help them unwind with a predictable and calming evening routine.

Chapter Eight

RELATIONSHIPS

Sheer logic suggests that the fact of being born a twin or a higher multiple would have an effect on many relationships and so it does, if only because there is someone else who is exactly the same age, making similar demands on parents. Also the number of children in a household makes the number of possible relationships within the family that much greater.

Most – maybe all – twins interact differently with those around them than would a singleton. Twins are not the same as one child, nor are they just two children very close in age. They are the same age: an obvious fact, but it is the crux of the problem. How does one deal with bed-time stories? Who goes first, leaving the other trailing in second?

> There'd be terrible trouble over who got kissed good night first. At two and a half, both boys would lie in bed calling out 'My arms are open.' I had to have a mental rota

Although twins tend to need the same things at the same time, it is not feasible for them to have them, so they have to learn to take turns, which some twins do at an earlier age than singletons. In the process of learning to do so, there is naturally a great deal of competition and rivalry between them. No wonder twins can develop intense and sometimes exclusive relationships.

· *Within the Twinship* ·

Love–hate is a good description for many twin relationships; good–bad is another. There are many positive aspects of twin relationships, such as:

- affection
- mutual support
- co-operation and encouragement
- stimulation
- sympathy
- empathy and understanding.

There are less attractive aspects, like:

- dominance or dependence
- competition
- collusion
- exclusivity.

It is, however, a bit simplistic to define characteristics in terms of good versus bad. Both positive and negative features may just be different expressions of the same phenomenon, for instance when support and co-operation are carried to extremes, or directed in less acceptable ways, the result may be little short of aiding and abetting.

> I doubt if at the age of three Oliver could have got the bucket stuck around his chest, but with Anthony's assistance he managed it. However, neither of them could get it off again. He was stuck, with the handle round the front and the pail part of the bucket sticking out of his back. Both were giggling helplessly. And so was I.

Identity

Twins usually spend more time together than they do with anyone else (including their mother), which is bound to be an important factor in the closeness and intensity of their relationship. Very early on, a twin may have difficulty in recognizing what is himself and what is not. The classical example of this is the identical twin looking into a mirror: is it himself or his twin he sees? If he is lying in a cot next to his twin and sucking a thumb, is it his own or his brother's? There can certainly be instances when twins seem to have just as much trouble as strangers have in telling each other apart. As the writer Mark Twain put it, 'When I was two weeks old my twin brother drowned in a bath, and to this day I don't know which one of us died.'

Nevertheless, we do have to learn to tell twins apart and so do they. Perhaps this is why twins often seem to allot each other different roles, so that they complement each other. At its most obvious, one may start a sentence and the other may finish it. One may make friends while the other remains in the background. One may try new things, whereas his twin does not, and so on. Professor René Zazzo, from France, calls such a division of labour between twins 'the couple effect'.

Couple effects may even mask or obscure genetic similarities. It is known that identical twins brought up together tend to be less alike than identicals brought up apart. Why? Perhaps it is because that's how the twins strive to be. Of course, parents influence their children too: adults probably both create and respond to any differences the children show. Many parents cherish and encourage their twins' dissimilarities. One could call these 'splitters'. There are also 'lumpers', parents who value their children's twin-ness above most other characteristics and tend to treat them as one unit.

While twins are growing up and learning to function independently of their mother, they have the extra task of growing away from each other. Dealing with twins as one unit can interfere with this process and cause long-term distress within a family (a topic explored in Chapter 15), but it is not at all unusual, especially when twins start coming into contact with more people outside the family, for instance at playgroup and school. On occasion outsiders may even refer to them as a singular noun, as in 'The twins is coming to the party.' This is not always a grammatical error – it is sometimes a slip of the mind.

Competition

Rivalry can be a good thing. Many parents comment that competition brings out the best in their twins, whether on the sports field or in the classroom. Your twins may even try to outdo each other by helping with household chores – if you are lucky.

> They'd both be champing at the bit, wanting to wash up or set the table, but as soon as one started helping me and showed he was enjoying it, the other would give up completely, find something else to do and simply fade into the background.

An element of competition and even conflict is normal. According to some psychiatrists and psychologists, trying to eliminate competition altogether could cause fresh problems within a family.

Of course, it can be unhealthy and lead to fighting, a topic covered in Chapter 9, which deals with behaviour and language. In any sort of battle, only one twin can win. This tends to accentuate any differences between them, with one taking up the leading role and the other following.

Some parents seem to mind this very much, believing that their twins should be strictly equal, while others are happy to acknowledge it openly in front of their children. 'His brother's the dominant one,' a mother may say without inhibition, though this could have an effect on the dependent twin's self-esteem and may stop him from ever trying to take the lead. You cannot entirely alter the balance of power within the twinship, but you can promote each child's individuality and sense of worth.

Comparison

To a certain extent, twins may enjoy being compared; after all this is one way in which they can assert their personalities. Comparisons can become invidious, however. One of the children may become the 'bad' one on a fairly permanent basis and end up as a scapegoat for everything that goes wrong. Sometimes parents or grandparents encourage this in subtle ways, either by saying, for example, 'It's always Katy' or just failing to express surprise when one twin in particular transgresses.

Obviously, nobody is ever wholly good or wholly bad and a good–bad split within the twinship is unfair. It gives neither child a chance. It's hard for the supposedly 'good' twin, who may have trouble living up to her halo, as well as for her sibling.

Scapegoating does of course happen in families without twins, but it is more awkward to handle when it involves children of the same age. One occasionally sees the reverse of this phenomenon, with one twin taking the rap for his twin's misbehaviour.

Understanding

Many, perhaps most, people assume that twins have some sort of tacit understanding and are able to share their feelings without verbal communication. Some twins seem to think so too. 'I don't need her to tell me anything when she's upset,' remarks one woman about her twin, 'I always know what's on Iris's mind.' 'Ask me – I always know what Oliver thinks,' says one seven-year-old boy.

A minimum of communication sometimes seems enough. For example, one mother took her one-year-old twin boys out shopping:

> I was in a bookshop with Alex and Kim facing each other in their pram. Alex made a few noises, Kim gurgled fluently in reply as if telling a joke and they were off in fits of giggles. It brought business in the shop to a standstill as people gawped.

Same-sex twins versus boy–girl pairs

It is generally agreed that identical twins tend to be the closest and most supportive of each other, even if they are sometimes bitter rivals. Boy twins have earned themselves something of a reputation for being a handful. Girl twins tend to be more biddable but can also be trouble. Girl twins, especially if identical and dressed in attractive matching outfits, often receive a great deal of admiration, and may get terribly blasé about being the centre of attention.

Non-identical twins can also be very close and some pairs are also very alike physically. Boy–girl pairs are perhaps the least similar, to look at anyway, and are sometimes not even considered to be 'real' twins. Among twins, their relationship tends to be the least exclusive, but it can still be very supportive. Often the girl is more advanced socially and physically and may take on the role of protector or 'mother' to her twin, something her brother may either enjoy or resent, especially if she bosses him about. The tables may turn in the teen years; this is discussed in later chapters.

The behaviour of boy–girl twins is often less stereotypical than it might have been had they been brother and sister born as singletons. The boy, for instance, may be gentler and less bellicose, something his parents may be grateful for.

Triplets

Three is an unstable number: many mothers comment that quads would have been less trouble. Although there are exceptions, triplets in many families don't seem to play well together all at the same time. One is often left out. This may either work on a sort of rota basis or with the same one of the three always being excluded, a situation which is hard to handle. An identical pair may cold-shoulder the third, non-identical member of their trio. Sometimes it is the one of different gender who is the odd one out; eventually he or she may come to detest being a triplet. This is an extremely difficult situation for a parent. All one can do is try to help each of the three develop as individuals and perhaps play down the significance of their triplet status.

· In the Womb ·

'They start as they mean to go on' is a warning many midwives give pregnant women who have a very active baby. Babies certainly have some life before birth, but what kind of life is it?

As young babies, twins play together from the age of a few months old, far sooner than do most singletons. It is now believed that some start interacting in the womb. There are known cases of triplets where one pair had very close contact before birth, kissing and stroking each other, while the third did not.

Some experts have speculated as to whether particular patterns of behaviour, or aspects of twin relationships, can be identified before birth. Alessandra Piontelli, an Italian psychoanalyst, recently studied twins antenatally with ultrasound and concluded that they interacted in such a way that they expressed their separate identities before birth.

She later studied the same children and found some surprising instances of continuity. For example, twin girls Marissa and Beatrice hit each other in the womb and did so after birth as soon as they were physically capable of it. Twins Alice and Luca stroked each other through the membrane that separated them and at the age of a year particularly enjoyed stroking each other from either side of a curtain. It is certainly tempting to make something of these observations, but the research was highly subjective (Piontelli studied the children herself both before and after birth) and nobody has yet managed to replicate its results on a more objective basis.

· *Birth Order* ·

Strangers often ask which twin is older: it's the most common question after 'Are they identical?' Before long, your children will be asking you too.

Unless you got them dreadfully shuffled in the ward and mislaid their plastic bracelets, at least you and your partner will know which twin was born first. But should you tell people?

While some parents are open with this information, others like to keep it to themselves and may not even tell their twins, at least not for a long time. The truth will out eventually. In the UK, the times of birth are given on multiples' birth certificates; hospital records and your GP's notes will also record the birth order. However, some parents prefer to keep it a family secret for a while. You can probably get away with telling the children themselves that they were born at exactly the same time, until, that is, they learn the mechanics of birth.

> Actually I told everyone they were born at the same time because I had a caesarean. Very few people outside medicine realize what happens at caesareans.

The trouble is that once you have spilled the beans, the news is out for good – but does it matter?

> Yes, it matters a lot, not to me but to my in-laws, who are Indian and regard the first-born boy as especially important. I hadn't realized it would be this way. If I had, I'd have kept it hushed up.

Rank is often important to an older sibling. Perhaps this is to be expected; after all, a big brother's status within the family depends crucially on the fact that he was born first. Once he knows the twins' birth order, he may accord the first-born much more seniority, or use it to explain different characteristics between the twins.

Often the first-born is indeed the dominant partner, though whether this is cause or effect is not certain. Research also suggests that the second-born twin often smiles more and is more eager to please. This applies especially to non-identicals of the same sex, but is by no means a universal rule.

Children can benefit from knowing their birth order. The shyer or more retiring twin may be delighted to learn that he was born first, ahead of his more assertive sibling.

Many twins like to know their birth order because it is the one thing they have which makes them different from each other. On the other hand, some regard it as unimportant. As one identical twin says:

> My brother and I came from the same egg. We were conceived at the same time and it is just a question of chance as to who poked his head out first.

Being the elder can be a disadvantage. Some people expect the first-born to be taller or more intelligent, as though a few minutes could really make much difference. Katya was older than her non-identical sister by eight minutes, which also made her the eldest of a family of six children. She knew this from an early age and it was a huge responsibility because she was expected to behave better.

Whether and when you tell your twins is up to you. On the whole, it is probably best to tell them in childhood rather than wait till the teen years or later, but the decision is yours.

> I could never bring myself to tell them because every time my girls asked who was born first, they were always in the middle of a flaming row and wanted to know just so they could decide how to settle the argument! It seemed the wrong moment when they were so het up, so I didn't tell them until they were nearly ten.

The elder may not always be the one you think: in some parts of Africa, the second twin is considered older, in fact senior enough to have ordered his twin out first to ensure the world was ready for him!

· *Favouritism* ·

You like Gareth more than me.

Having a favourite is very common, as mentioned in Chapter 4 ('Favourites', page 93). This is very natural and often sorts itself out. In time you may even find your preference reverses completely.

However, favouritism can persist and there may be lasting inequality in the feelings a parent has for the twins. If this is the case, ask yourself why you have a permanent favourite. Is it the first-born, or the boy of a boy–girl pair? Perhaps this is for stereotypical reasons, which may do both your twins a disservice.

Is your favourite child achieving more? This could be one effect as well as the cause of your feelings. If so, try to help the less able twin achieve his potential. He may not even be significantly less able: parents frequently exaggerate minute differences and ignore the fact that twins are often more similar to each other than to anyone else on earth.

What should you do if you have a favourite?

- First of all, don't feel guilty. This only makes things worse. As the family therapist Audrey Sandbank says, it is important not to get too hung up about favouritism.

- We all like some things more than others. Accept your current feelings as a fact of life, but avoid dwelling on them or making them too public, especially in front of the children.

- Do your best to avoid labelling and comparing. Labels change.

- Try to act fairly, however hard this is. Fair is not necessarily equal. A naughty child should not go unpunished, nor a good child unrewarded, just because he has a twin.

- Don't overcompensate. If you try to make it up to the less favoured one, you may reinforce unacceptable behaviour and make him even less favoured!

- It may not be you who has a favourite, but someone else, like your partner, a grandparent or a child-minder. It does happen. In this situation it is very important to be fair and get all the adults concerned to consider the points listed above; otherwise you could end up with alliances being forged. This can set the whole family at odds and also make discipline very tricky.

· *Relationships with Siblings* ·

It is hard being the brother or sister of a set of twins. Australian research suggests that 64 per cent of families with young twins have problems with the older child. This seems to be the case especially when there are identical twins in the family, perhaps because there is too much emphasis (from the older child's point of view) on twin-ness.

Being between eighteen months and three years of age when twins are born seems to be particularly difficult, and no wonder. A toddler is old enough to appreciate what is going on, but too young to accept it without a fight. Look at the situation from his point of view and imagine what it is like to be upstaged by not one new arrival, but two.

Babies take up your time, energy and both your arms, all of which the older child still needs. The twins will probably sleep in your bedroom for a month or more. Meanwhile logistics may mean that your toddler must move into a big bed now, or start walking because you cannot push his buggy as well as a twin pram. And all this around the time he starts potty-training or going to playgroup.

Whenever someone comes round, or stops to chat in the street, you can bet that all the attention is focused on the twins, with the older child being either ignored or asked how he likes being a big brother now. He may be expected suddenly to 'be big', but he doesn't know how and may not want to anyway. In fact it might be nicer to be a twin too. Some children revert to bed-wetting at this stage, or to temper tantrums. Others – boys included – enjoy having a doll to be their twin for a while, or invent an imaginary twin.

The jealous older sibling may indulge in attention-seeking behaviour of any type and become aggressive towards the twins. This is very stressful to a parent already at the end of her tether; some researchers have reported a higher incidence of child abuse in the siblings of twins.

Eventually all may be well. In later years your older child may get on famously with one of the twins, or else function happily on his own or relate to a younger child (if you have any more). Some children will have lasting difficulties. Audrey Sandbank points out that siblings of twins need family therapy more often than twins themselves. The use of 'he' in the above is deliberate: compared with girls, boys seem to find it harder to adapt to younger multiples in the family. Audrey Sandbank suggests this is because young girls can remain in centre stage more easily, and also because they continue to have much the same relationship with their father.

· *Helping the Older Sibling* ·

The earlier you start thinking about how your older child may feel, the more you can do to ease things for him.

Before the twins are born

- Don't tell him about the pregnancy too soon. Six or eight months is a long time to a toddler so you may as well wait till your bump shows, but do answer his questions. He won't like being left in the dark or having to piece together what is happening from overheard snippets of conversation.

- Avoid telling him the babies are just for him. They won't be much use as playmates for years to come. In fact, he may find them rather boring.

- Nor should you tell him he's getting twins because he's been so good. It is possible that there will be complications, for which he may then blame himself.

- Avoid moaning about your symptoms, even if you have a more troublesome pregnancy this time around. It could bias him against the twins from an early stage.

- Make him feel special, but don't expect him to be too grown-up. He may find it daunting if you tell him you will need his help with the babies: he's far too young for parental responsibilities! But you could explain that you will still want all his love and hugs (and vice versa).

- If there is plenty of time left and you were about to potty-train him, start him at playgroup or move him to a big bed, go ahead. It is best not to do these immediately before or after the twins are born.

- Try to find him a special older person to relate to, some-one who will make a bit of a fuss of him. It could be an aunt, uncle, godparent, teenaged neighbour – anyone trustworthy whom he likes and who can be relied on to give him time and attention. These commodities will be in short supply when the babies arrive.

- If he has been going to a child-minder and likes her, consider letting this continue if you can, perhaps for a couple of hours every so often. The contact may help him.

When they arrive

- Someone your child likes (and you trust) is obviously the best person to look after him when you are in hospital.

- Let him come to the hospital to see the babies. Again, avoid moaning about your stitches or your symptoms.

- When you ring home, ask to speak to your son on the phone.

- Let him choose (even if it's with your money) something for the babies to have in their cots, maybe their first small soft toy. Tell him he can also decide who should get which.

- Encourage him to touch the babies if he wants to. You may need to show him how to be gentle, as you would if you had just got a tiny kitten.

- Consider getting a special present for him.

When you get home

Many toddlers seem to take this stage very well, but sibling rivalry and regressive behaviour don't necessarily manifest themselves immediately.

> I really thought Thomas was fine. He was interested in the twins, sweet-natured and acting perfectly normally, so I thought, 'no problem'. It wasn't until they were about six weeks old that he changed completely. He became very aggressive, wouldn't eat, wouldn't sleep and started wetting himself, which he carried on doing for nearly a year. I was at the end of my tether with three of them in nappies.

Not every toddler reacts like this, but it is probably safe to assume that your older child's nose will be put slightly out of joint when the twins physically invade his home.

- Make time for him. If you have help, and your twins are fit and well, consider using it for the babies, so that you can devote yourself to your older child. Parents who have done this say it was the right thing to do and would definitely adopt the same strategy again.

- Allow him to stay up later than the babies if possible. This may be hard on you at first, but he'll appreciate it.

- You may be exhausted, but try not to shout at your child.

- Give him plenty of cuddles and reassurance.

- Praise him whenever possible. He may be feeling negative at the moment, but you should try not to be!

- Some older siblings, whether boys or girls, are ready and willing to assist with bathing, feeding, etc., but many are not and may resent feeling they have to. Give your older child the chance to get involved, but don't push him into it.

- Think about giving him a doll or teddy to change or feed while you look after the babies. He may discard it after a while, but it can help during the first few months. This is a poor time, however, for getting a family pet, as some parents learn the hard way.

- You are at your most vulnerable when feeding both babies at once, with no spare hands. This may be a good time to get out something special for him, whether it is a favourite video, a new jigsaw puzzle or just a cardboard box full of safe but interesting junk. This could turn into a useful ritual at feeding-time.

- When people turn up and coo at the babies or stop you in the street and peek into the pram, make sure your toddler is not left out. If you are asked what the babies are called, for instance, introduce your older child first; make a point of including him.

- Give your older child his own space and make sure his toys can go somewhere they won't be damaged by the babies, especially once they start chewing, dribbling, crawling and going on the rampage.

- Continue with his usual routine, such as bedtime stories, for as long as possible.

- Give him special outings on his own. He will have to get used to the new arrivals being part of the family, but all in due time.

- It could be a good idea to start giving him weekly pocket money, but don't go overboard to compensate or give him a lot of sweets, crisps or things you might regret later.

- Don't leave him on his own with the twins. At this stage he may be less reliable than the family dog.

- If he is threatening to (or has already) hurt the babies, explain that he shouldn't, and try to give him an incentive to behave better in future. If he doesn't poke the babies' eyes all morning, he might be read a story, for instance. Reward systems can be very effective.

· Siblings of Triplets or More ·

The arrival of triplets or quads is particularly tough on an older child. Apart from the fact that you will be extra busy, triplets are sufficiently unusual to ensure that they hog all the attention from friends and strangers, and sometimes from the media too.

Again, make a point of introducing your older child – in his own right not as 'the triplets' brother', and include him in any photos, whether they are for the family album or for publicity.

If you give any interviews to the Press, make sure your older child gets a mention. In general, it is always a good idea to get the journalist's name and phone number in case you have any further thoughts before an article goes to press. You could even ask to see the piece to check it before it is published. Think carefully about what you say. An older child can be acutely embarrassed when personal details appear in the local paper. You may be, too. Remember, neighbours and friends may read what is published and you will have to live with it. Don't say anything you would mind seeing in print, for instance whether you had fertility treatment.

You may not get any fees for interviews and appearances, but it doesn't hurt to ask. Make sure you are not out of pocket: reimbursement of expenses is normal. You could give your older child a small slice of the money.

· *Parents and Twins* ·

When you become a parent you have to revise your own view of yourself – certainly most other people see women differently once they are mothers – and your life-style changes are likely to be far more dramatic when two or more babies arrive at once.

As a mother of twins, you will be busier than other mothers and will have to shift your attention more often from one child to the other. The relationship between the twins themselves will also affect how you relate to them: they may appear to need your approval less than a singleton might, for instance. Your feelings towards them could also be influenced by the fact that more people, whether from your extended family or from an *au pair* agency, may be involved in their care. For all these reasons, mothers sometimes relate differently to twins than they might have done to two singletons.

> I don't think I ever felt Alex and Kim really needed me, unlike my first son. The twins always seemed self-sufficient, and once they were about two or three years old they almost excluded me. I'd take them to the park and instead of being with them and pointing things out to them they'd toddle off happily together.

The experience of another mother was entirely different.

> Having twin daughters took me completely by surprise and I thought I'd never get used to it. I didn't want to breast-feed them, unlike my older daughter, whom I breast-fed for six months. But funnily I am much closer to the twins than to my first child. And they are more affectionate towards me. Perhaps it breaks all the rules, but there it is.

There is no such thing as a typical mother, nor are there typical twins, so it's doubtful whether there are any useful blanket rules that govern the relationships of mothers and their twins. One important generalization, though, is that the less happy you were to be pregnant with twins, the more trouble you may later have relating to them. That's one very good reason to get as much psychological and practical support as you need before they arrive.

· *The Parents as a Couple* ·

What happens to the parents themselves? In a family with twins, fathers often make a much more active contribution than usual. One of the pluses of having multiples is that it opens a new dimension for a father and gives him the chance of doing some hands-on parenting. When they are needed, the least promising men sometimes turn into the most adept fathers. Unfortunately, the opposite can happen too.

Multiples make a family special. Men often enjoy boasting about being the father of twins or triplets. In many ways, multiples can draw a family closer (rather like wars do), because you are all in it together, but for some couples twins are the last two nails in the marital coffin.

Parents argue most often about children and money, and having young multiples will provide many occasions to row about both. The odds are particularly stacked against those for whom the pregnancy was unplanned, who already had at least one child under the age of two, or who have triplets or more. Mothers often find that identical twins and twin boys, whether identical or not, impose particular strains on a marriage.

One father of twins, an architect, commented:

> Le Corbusier said a house was a machine for living in. Well, if you asked me what a couple was for, for years I'd have said it was a machine for raising children. A very efficient machine, I might add, but that's all it did. After having twins there was nothing left in either my wife or myself for each other.

Twins tend to dominate a family, not only getting most of the attention but also dictating what can and cannot be done. Fathers and other siblings may be squeezed out of the wife's timetable by the constant demands of caring for multiples. A mother especially can wear herself out trying to be a perfect parent and home-maker (as Americans call it). Tiredness may be extreme, money short and leisure activities dropped because they become impractical. It is harder to go out in the evenings: can next door's young teenager cope with baby-sitting two or three small children?

One's horizons can soon shrink, isolating a family socially, and sex may become a chore. It is far healthier to take the long view of parenting, which is that you, as a couple, are important too. After all, children grow up eventually and you and your partner will have to survive after the kids have left home.

There are no sure-fire ways of keeping romance or lust alive, or of ensuring you stay the course together, but the following suggestions have worked for many parents.

- Go out together once in a while. It needn't be expensive if you join a baby-sitting circle. I know many mothers of twins who did not go out for two years or more after their children were born. When they finally did, some wondered just who was this person they married. 'I recognized him, of course,' one of them joked. 'He was the bloke I used to meet at 3 am traipsing the corridor with a crying baby.'

- Join your local twins' club. Apart from some of the social activities you may be interested in taking part in, it will demonstrate that there is indeed life after twins.

- Try not to argue over trivia. It is just not worth it. If you really feel like exploding over the dirty socks in the hall (again) why not just say, 'I really feel like exploding'?

- Every so often, have a candle-lit dinner. It can be in your own kitchen, but the point is that the atmosphere must be relaxing and make a contrast from the usual run of meals eaten on the hop.

- Pretend you've only just met your partner. This sounds stupid and it may not work for you, but many couples find it quite exciting to have to start at the beginning with each other, flirting and thinking of loving, sexy things to say.

- Try spending a whole evening (or however long you have) stroking each other everywhere but the genitals. Many people are driven to distraction by this arousal technique, which is used in some kinds of sex therapy. (There is a poignant description of it in David Lodge's 1991 novel *Paradise News*.)

- Get some reliable contraception. It is said that young babies are in themselves a method of birth control, but alas, they arc not. Women who have twins are often more fertile, and it is not unknown for a second set of twins to be born within a year or so. Even if you are not one of these lucky few, you don't want to lie awake at night worrying whether you are pregnant with triplets. There is no ideal contraceptive. Choose one that seems effective enough for you without having an unacceptable level of side-effects (if any). Don't put off your decision.

Chapter Nine

BEHAVIOUR AND LANGUAGE

'Twins! How lovely!' This may be what a lot of people say, but these aren't exactly the words most likely to trip off your tongue when your twins act up – and they will. When they do, you will probably see why, in some African tribes, 'May you be the mother of twins' is considered to be one of the worst possible curses.

> We went for the day to my in-laws. Martha and David were two years old. In under three hours they'd stamped on the video, unplugged all the appliances, forcibly taken the aerial out of the telly, broken an antique clock and torn wallpaper off the wall. They ended the afternoon by squabbling under the dining-table.

All children fight, don't they? Of course they do. But research shows that bad – or, if you prefer, socially imma-ture – behaviour is about twice as common in twins aged three than it is in singletons. More to the point, perhaps, some parents know from experience that twins can be very hard to control, occasionally to the point where they exhaust all concerned. In a small number of cases, there is a connec-tion between language and behaviour difficulties, which is why this chapter deals with both.

· *Bad Behaviour* ·

There is evidence that:

- temper tantrums (see Chapter 7) tend to go on past the stage when most singletons grow out of them
- twins tend to lack concentration
- bad behaviour is generally more common in school-age twins, especially identical boys.

The fact that misbehaviour is more common in twins doesn't mean that yours will be a handful and certainly not that they will be non-stop terrors.

> My two boys were lovely at least 90 per cent of the time. It is just that in the other 10 per cent, when they 'went ballistic', I'd be at my wits' end. Often I couldn't guess in advance when it would be, though looking back – the boys are now ten – I remember that they were most likely to act up when I was making an important phone call. They'd usually just shout, or else fight, and once Kim pushed Alex through a glass door.

· *Why do Multiples Misbehave?* ·

It is difficult to pinpoint just one cause since so many factors can operate in the misbehaviour of multiples. Here are some of the most important:

- Twins and more compete fiercely for your time. What surer way of getting attention than to behave badly (as some adult celebrities demonstrate)?

- Twins often co-operate or collude. They egg each other on, are physically able to cause more trouble and may cover up for each other. Under these circumstances even very experienced parents can find it difficult to discipline twins.

- Because they communicate with each other, they simply may not listen to anyone else. What does eventually get through (your shouting, for instance) tends to be very confrontational.

- They have each other and therefore may feel less in need of adult approval. Some parents take this in their stride, without fully realizing it, but once the twins start school, teachers can find it very obvious.

- Male twins tend to have less contact with their mother and less affection shown to them than to two-year-old singleton boys. It is not known why this happens, but research shows that it does, and it might be significant.

- It is physically harder to restrain two or more children who misbehave, especially on outings.

- Some twins have delayed language development (dealt with later in this chapter), which is occasionally linked with difficult behaviour. It is not necessarily so, however; there are badly behaved twins without any language problems at all. In fact, there can be a marked disparity between how well they speak and read and how appallingly they sometimes act!

- If you are a single parent, establishing discipline becomes even more of a challenge. It is more difficult to be firm without another adult to back you up, though one obvious plus is that you don't have another adult disagreeing with your methods.

- When one child has special needs, it is hard to know just how much discipline is right. In setting boundaries shouldn't one take into account his individual problems and not be too strict? On the other hand, the healthy twin also has needs and she may perceive her parents to be grossly unfair (there is more on this situation in Chapter 14).

- Australian research shows that a number of twins have attention deficit hyperactivity disorder (ADHD), which significantly affects concentration and learning. Having studied 2300 families, Professor David Hay found that ADHD is almost twice as common in twins as in singletons and affects 16 per cent of boy twins and 8 per cent of girl twins. There's more on ADHD in the Appendix (page 335).

· *Pre-empting Problems* ·

Discipline may seem an ugly word, but it is an essential part of child-rearing and all children have to learn it. In a nutshell, these are the most important things you can do to get the best from your twins:

- aid their individual development (sometimes called 'individuation')
- give your attention fairly
- handle them consistently
- set a good example.

There are many different strategies and steps which can help you, and you will no doubt have ideas which suit your own circumstances. The following advice has worked well for many parents of multiples:

- Try to be fair but firm. If you don't normally allow the children to get down from table without asking, don't make exceptions.

- Make sure you address each twin. How can a child respond appropriately if he doesn't know who's being asked to put on his shoes?

- Try to give the same amount of attention to each, if necessary using the kitchen timer to be – and be seen to be – scrupulously fair.

- Give each child a chance to have his say with you in private, for instance at bathtime or bedtime. Privacy is something multiples rarely get.

- Separate outings can be an eye-opener. If one of your little monsters becomes delightful on his own, then that, says twins expert Dr Elizabeth Bryan, is how he really is.

- Do your best to be positive rather than negative. A child would rather hear 'Do go with Grandpa' rather than 'Don't be such a slowcoach.'

- Some sort of challenge or dare can help. An incredulous 'Can you really do your shoes?' may work wonders, as can 'Bet you can't put the bricks away in two minutes.'

- Try to set boundaries – reasonable ones! It is pointless being obsessional about, say, tidiness when you have several young children.

- Give simple reasons for your rules whenever you can. Being rushed, mothers of twins tend to issue only short instructions, but 'Just because' is maddening to children.

- Try not to let them get bored or overtired as they will be more difficult to handle.

- Make sure you know when they are ill. Normally kids are naughtier far more often than they are unwell, but even parents who are doctors or nurses occasionally get caught out.

- If you are at the end of your tether or unwell yourself, don't be too ambitious with activities. Scrap the trip to the supermarket if you can and just try to get through the day doing the minimum in a low-key way.

- Keep temptation away where possible. For instance, put cherished objects out of reach. And if you never put 20p in one of those Postman Pat machines children ride in the shopping centre, your children won't act up on the occasions when you refuse to.

- Stay in control yourself. Shouting unnecessarily just cranks up the aggression; besides it makes you a poor role model.

- If you threaten your children, it has to be with something you would actually carry out. They will soon realize that you won't dump them on the dual carriageway if they scream in the car or get the neighbour's child in to finish their meals when they don't eat up.

- Try not to use food (or lack of it) as a punishment. It only makes meals more emotionally charged.

- Get help before a real crisis occurs. A friend who takes just one of the children for a couple of hours could defuse an explosive situation.

- If you have one, a responsible older child is a useful ally, but beware the big brother or sister who just likes bossing the little ones about.

- Always praise your children on the rare occasions when they admit to a misdemeanour. Owning up is a particular problem with young twins and they certainly won't do it if it results in punishment.

- Whatever has happened during the day, try not to put them to bed on a bad note. Kissing and making up makes for sweeter dreams.

· *Coping with Wayward Twins* ·

All the way home, they were hitting each other in the back of the car with the book I'd just borrowed from the library – it happened to be *Toddler Taming* . . . .

Identical twin boys tend to mature most slowly and have earned a reputation for having the biggest behaviour problems. They may need a particularly firm, but loving, hand. Many mothers have found that separate bedrooms are warranted on the basis of their lack of discipline when together, but don't be too surprised if, having moved to a larger house, they spend a lot of time in each other's bedrooms! (As well as arguing frequently about the size of their respective rooms.)

Whatever your type of twins or triplets, they will inevitably have their trying moments. In time you will evolve your own personal style of dealing with these, but meanwhile the following advice will help:

- When your twins are naughty, express disapproval of what they did but assure them you still love them (e.g. 'I love you but I hate what you just did to your sister').

- Make the bad behaviour seem really boring. You may need to separate warring twins (more on this later), but giving the aggressor attention can reinforce bad behaviour.

- Don't smack, unless perhaps there is physical danger, such as when a child fiddles with the oven door or runs into the road.

- Get them to apologize whenever one has been tormenting the other(s). A churlishly mumbled 'Sorry' may be all you get. Well, you cannot expect miracles.

- Say sorry yourself when you get things wrong. It sets a good example. Besides, being fallible can excuse your mistakes in future . . . .

- Try to avoid making one child a scapegoat, even if it is consistently one of your twins who misbehaves. When you are not sure who did a dirty deed, you can either let both off (which encourages collusion), or else punish both (this is unfair, but if you choose a relatively mild and reversible punishment it can work well and some parents find it also helps twins own up).

- 'Time out' in another room, or spent standing in the corner, has become a time-honoured method of discipline and usefully separates warring twins, but in the very young it only works when used for short periods of time, say five minutes for a five-year-old. The idea is not for the child to find something more interesting to do (or mischief to create), but to remove him from the scene of the crime. Of course there will be times when you want them to play separately for 45 minutes at a stretch, but it is best for it not to be a punishment.

- It is not a good idea to send one twin up to his bedroom too often: he may end up disliking his bedroom, and bedtime. Also, the one who is left playing downstairs may gloat – unfairly, if they've both been naughty. When twins share a bedroom, sending them both upstairs is obviously counter-productive.

· *Special Problems* ·

Should you stop them fighting?

Twins often fight, as the rhyme about Tweedledum and Tweedledee suggests. When mine were locked in battle, my thoughts would turn to the teenaged Ronnie and Reggie Kray, who used to entertain East Enders by fighting in the ring.

Fighting passes eventually and well-adjusted young adult twins rarely come to blows, but it can seem an eternity until then. As one mother says:

> The boys are nine and a half now and most days I still cannot go and have a bath in peace, or even use the loo, without World War III breaking out. Last time, one tried to strangle the other with his school tie.

The cause is not often aggression in itself. School-age twins – including the ones just mentioned – may fight each other in the playground as well as at home on a daily basis, yet hardly lay a finger on their classmates.

The big question is whether or not to intervene. Those who have singletons tend to advise other parents to let the children get on with it, but you often get a different point of view from mothers of twins who have ended up in Casualty from wounds inflicted on each other. Even hospital treatment may not inhibit twins from giving each other near-mortal blows for long.

The issue of fighting multiples is far from straightforward, and methods which work with aggressive singletons may not work with twins. One mother had difficulties with her three-year-old boys, one of whom had been hitting his twin on the head with a stick. When she removed the stick, the offender cried bitterly and the victim was so moved that he retrieved the stick and returned it to his brother, whereupon the violence began anew!

One characteristic of fighting twins – or triplets – is that when they fight they do so without any inhibitions or self-restraint, causing far worse injuries than a singleton would inflict on a friend or sibling. Perhaps serious fighting breaks out because both are at a similarly immature stage of development. Their lack of control may also relate to their earliest days as babies, when they hardly realized where the body of one of them stopped and the other's began.

At one point, driven to distraction by their frequent screams and punch-ups, I asked each of my own boys, then aged eight, whether they thought a grown-up should stop one of their fights. Without hesitating, each said that I should. But they couldn't offer any hints as to how I might actually achieve this . . . .

As for the tactics you should adopt, most parents of twins who have gone through this phase advise playing things by ear. Letting them get on with it and sort them-selves out is fine if nobody is getting hurt, and if there are no potentially lethal weapons lying about. Under these circumstances they may well work it out of their systems within a couple of minutes and once again become the best of friends. But it is useful to keep an ear out for signs that things are getting too rough, so that you can intervene before they reach the stage of GBH.

Biting

> The first two-word phrase one of my twins strung together was an indignant 'Bit me!'

> My girls were very pretty as toddlers, or would have been had they not given each other nasty bites on such a regular basis. This could be anywhere on the body, including their faces. As the teethmarks faded, they'd look like bruises, and I'm sure passers-by wondered what I'd been doing to them.

One of the most frequent problems brought to both TAMBA and MBF is that of biting two-year-olds. Audrey Sandbank and Dr Elizabeth Bryan warn parents that giving the perpe-trator attention is often the last thing they ought to do. One mother, for example, resorted to carrying her two-year-old son constantly to prevent him biting the other two triplets. He thereby gained exactly what he wanted.

Biting tends to be restricted to the twin or triplet group; they rarely bite other children. Often both twins bite each other, though in any given incident there is usually a perpetrator and a victim. Handling biting toddlers is tricky because they can do so much damage unchecked – and incidentally teeth carry bacteria.

The best method of dealing with an attack of biting is simply to remove the offender and give him minimal atten-tion, to make the biting seem really boring and unrewarding. Whatever you do, don't let him see that his behaviour riles you.

TAMBA's consultant family therapist, Audrey Sandbank, particularly recommends picking up the victim and giving him two minutes of undivided attention. If the biter interrupts, explain that, because he was biting, he has to wait. He'll soon get the idea.

Should you bite back? Some mothers advocate this, but it rarely works and often makes matters worse. If anything, it suggests to youngsters that violence in general and biting in particular are acceptable within the family.

· *Getting Help for Behaviour* · *Problems*

There are several avenues of help for established problems, including:

- your GP or health visitor: they are unlikely to be experienced in dealing with multiples, but can still give useful advice and support and make appropriate referrals to other agencies.

- TAMBA Twinline: you can discuss your difficulties with trained volunteers who are themselves parents of twins or more. TAMBA also has honorary consultants who may be able to help.

- MBF Clinics: telephone consultations can help, or your children may need to be seen in the clinic, for which a referral letter is needed either from your GP or Social Services.

- Family Guidance Therapy: usually available locally (your GP can refer you). As Audrey Sandbank points out, this is an excellent method for twins and results can often be seen quite quickly. It works best when started early, preferably before age five, but there are no firm rules on this.

- An educational psychologist: especially if there are problems in school-age twins (discuss referral with your children's teacher). Difficulties at school need not be educational in nature for the child to qualify for being seen by an educational psychologist – they can be primarily behavioural or social problems.

- The Maudsley Hospital Children's Department in London has a clinic for twins and higher multiples up to sixteen years old who have behavioural or emotional problems. You will need referral from your GP, hospital consultant or social worker.

(For addresses and telephone numbers of the above, see Resources, page 343.)

· *Language* ·

Even back in the 1930s, it was known that the language of twins at ages two, three, four and five was subtly different from that of singletons. Since then, a great deal of research, including work from Australia, has confirmed this and has helped piece together a picture of language development in twins. There has been far less work done on triplets and more – most of this section is therefore about twins.

Language is a set of symbols for communicating thought and can be written or spoken. Of course, children usually learn to speak before they read or write, so a child's acquisition of language generally refers to speech and how it is used. Acquiring language is a twofold process: understanding others and producing speech.

How do children learn language? Although experts debate the relative importance of various aspects, major factors include:

- a child's innate readiness or ability
- intelligence, or understanding of the world
- imitation.

This last factor should not be underestimated. I well remember the mother who brought her child to the paediatric clinic because he hardly spoke. ''Course,' she added, 'he can say "Bugger off".'

With twins, the general trend is that:

- twins are older than singletons when they say their first word
- the length of each utterance is shorter
- sentence structure is simpler
- vocabulary is smaller
- baby-talk persists longer.

On average, twins are about six months behind singletons in language development. This is not to imply that all twins fall behind singletons. Many twins are very advanced in their use of language and, just because research highlights the ones who aren't, it doesn't mean your children will have problems.

There is still a lot of work going on this area and the last word on language has yet to be spoken. One huge current project is the Twins' Early Development Study (TEDS). If your twins were born in England or Wales during 1994, 1995 or 1996 you may already have been invited to take part in this study, which looks at language and its interplay with other characteristics, such as behaviour and genetics.

· *Problems* ·

Does it matter if your twins' language is delayed? It is now becoming clear that language difficulties are often transient. In other words, they are a delay, not a disorder. In most twins, language delay has no long-term consequences for their education or their behaviour.

All the same, it is important for parents and teachers to be aware of possible language difficulties because:

- there is sometimes a link between poor language development and bad behaviour, especially in twin boys
- some twins with language problems early on will have trouble reading
- help can be given; it works best if started early
- good use of words is an essential part of success in other areas.

At school, many subjects, even Maths, depend heavily on word power. A child with language difficulties is not necessarily stupid or 'slow', but his score in IQ tests may well be misleadingly low until his problems are overcome.

Reasons for language problems

The fact that a parent of twins cannot give each child undivided attention probably lies at the root of language delay, just as it does of many other difficulties in twins. Singletons from large families also tend to have fewer verbal skills, so perhaps the situation of twins is an extreme example of the same phenomenon.

When the language skills of twins are studied closely, it is found that there is one thing they are very good at: responding quickly, though not necessarily to their mother! When the pressure is on, one obviously becomes adept at getting a word in.

Research and observations show the challenges that parents and their twins face and some of the reasons for language problems:

- Constant interruptions mean that mothers of young twins are less able to have long conversations or interactions with their children.

- Mothers of twins tend to talk in simpler, shorter sentences. It is obvious, perhaps, that with two toddlers you are more likely to say urgently, 'Put that down!' rather than patiently explain, 'Now, that's a very pretty vase that Mummy and Daddy got as a present, and we don't want you to break it.'

- Mothers tend to talk to both children at the same time. In 'Paul-and-James come here' neither Paul nor James is spoken to as an individual. Much of the day's conversation may be in this form.

- Because of rivalry and lack of privacy, many of the conversations a mother has with each of her twins are really three-way events, so-called 'triadic communication', a confusing exchange similar to talking on the phone while someone else is also taking part on another extension.

- When a mother speaks to one twin, her gestures and actions may, confusingly, have nothing to do with what she's saying. When you next feed your youngsters, for instance, you may notice that you are spooning food into one while carrying on an unrelated patter with the other baby.

- Mothers tend to respond less to multiples – after all, it is easy to assume they can keep each other company.

- It is not quite clear why, but two-year-old boy twins may be spoken to less by their parents – and even seem to get fewer hugs than singletons. Many mothers reckon they shout more at their boys, though.

- Twins tend to understand each other's needs and can communicate with body language, so it may be less important for them to speak aloud to each other. This probably applies most to identical (MZ) twins.

- When twins talk, they often make the same mistakes as each other, which reinforces errors and may even worsen them. Research shows that young twins aged two to four understand each other's speech well, even when it is full of mispronunciations. This doesn't happen with other children of the same age.

- Mothers may not bother to correct twins' inaccurate speech as much as they might a singleton's. It is partly pressure of time, but baby-talk can be attractive. As Audrey Sandbank points out, some mothers find it part of the undeniable 'cuteness' of young twins.

- Triplet language difficulties tend to be similar to those of twins, though they may perhaps be slightly worse. It seems to depend on how much external help is available to the family and how much individual attention the children get. However, it is hard to generalize; those who treat triplets with language disorders inevitably see a small pre-selected group.

- Finally, prematurity, growth retardation in the womb, birth difficulties and genetic influences can all have a bearing on language problems. These can affect singletons too. In fact recent work by Dr Dorothy Bishop in Cambridge demonstrates the likelihood that significant language impairment in twins has the same sorts of causes as in single-born children.

· How to Encourage Language · Development

Perhaps you cannot do much about prematurity or any medical complications your twins may have already had as newborns, but there are still plenty of factors you can influence in your children's early life to help avoid language problems. There is no evidence that twins with language or speech delay have any difficulty with comprehension. This suggests that in most cases the potential is there and all one need do is exploit it.

Some of the points below were highlighted by the La Trobe Twin Study in Australia and are widely accepted as important.

- Although it has not been conclusively proven, it appears that, starting from the tender age of four months, encouragement from parents can help develop language skills later. Here is where time and attention, including the all-important eye contact, really matter. Spending time with the babies and talking to them individually is not only more enjoyable than doing chores – it pays off. When speaking to them, make sure your actions match your words.

- When your twins start to speak, get them to talk to express what they want. Life may be more peaceful if you continue to anticipate their needs, as when they were tiny, but this will not teach them to communicate. If one will only point at his cup and grunt, you could say 'You want milk?' In time, this will encourage him to use words.

- Let each child speak for herself. One twin shouldn't talk for the other. Try to ask each about, for instance, how playgroup was that morning. At first they will no doubt argue over who should have her say first, but they eventually learn to take turns when answering questions.

- Don't put up with interruptions or attention-seeking behaviour. A good start is to ignore interruptions, and of course not to do it yourself. (Easier said than done.)

- Show them what good speech sounds like, without making a big issue of it, or saying, 'No, it is supposed to be . . . '. Just repeat, in its correct form, the word your child has pronounced wrongly. The message will get through.

- If baby-talk persists, encourage them to realize that speaking better will help them communicate better with others, get what they want more easily, make more friends and so on. This is tough, because many grown-ups find lisping attractive. Your efforts at promoting good speech may be undermined by people who smile and laugh at your children's most immature utterances.

- Read to each child separately from an early age. If you can manage it, ten uninterrupted minutes a day for each twin can work wonders. It is far better to do this than to read to both simultaneously for twenty minutes. The difficulty is that you need someone else – another adult or an older child – to keep one twin amused and out of the way. Of course it is nice to sit with a child tucked under each arm, so there is no reason why you shouldn't read to both together as well, if you have time.

- An older child can be useful as a role model, but only if his speech is good. It is often pointless to rely on a sibling who is only a bit older than the twins: apart from any rivalry which may exist, he too may have language difficulties, which will only compound the twins' problems.

- Watch out too for the older sister or brother who may dote on the twins and gratify all their needs, which sometimes happens. However convenient this may be for you, it probably won't help the youngsters' development.

· *Language Development* ·

It is not always easy to know when there are real difficulties. Some language problems, such as a slight delay, vanish in time, while others need treatment.

An added complication is that normal children vary: they don't all learn to speak at the same age, though on the whole they do develop speech in a predetermined order.

In the first eight weeks of life, babies make basic noises like crying and straining. From two to six months, there is usually laughter, cooing and chuckling, often in response to what the mother does or says.

The stage between six and twelve months is sometimes called vocal play. Babies enjoy making sounds and begin to babble. Towards the end of the first year words are finally produced – just single syllables to start with, and often the same sound for different things. At this stage one may notice that babies with different mother tongues begin to make slightly different noises.

Between eighteen months and two years, sentences are formed and they gradually increase in complexity. Much of grammar is probably acquired by the age of five.

Sounds are not all equally easy to produce. They tend to appear in this order:

Normally, by this age	. . . these sounds are no problem:
1^1/$_2$ years	p, b, m, h, w
2^1/$_2$ years	t, d, n, k, g, gn
3 years	y, f, s
4 years	sh, z, v
5 years	ch, j, l
7 years	th, r

There are differences from culture to culture. For instance some sounds which are perfectly easy for, say, five-year-old Arabic speakers can still pose a huge challenge for English speakers at any age!

Spotting problems

The following checklist, drawn from Adelaide Hospital and the La Trobe study, is a useful guide to spotting problems. You should suspect speech difficulties if one or both your twins shows any of these symptoms:

- is more than a year late mastering the sounds listed above
- uses mainly vowel sounds when speaking
- speaks unintelligibly after two and a half years of age
- leaves out or substitutes consonants after the age of three
- distorts lots of consonants after the age of four
- talks with an odd rhythm or unusual pitch (e.g. monoto nous, nasal, or too loud).

Other symptoms of language disorder include:

- not 'playing' with words by the age of one
- no spoken words by the age of one and a half
- no two-word phrases by two years of age
- no sentences by the age of three, or only sentences which are echoes of what the child hears
- baby-talk or very poor sentence structure after the age of four.

If a child has trouble with sentence construction as well as with making sounds and interpreting meaning, there is like-ly to be a significant problem that needs treatment.

What you can do

The linguist David Crystal believes that by the age of seven or eight, the language delay of twins, often very obvious at the age of three, will have disappeared. This seems to be confirmed by others in the field – as long as the delay is fairly mild.

There are a few twins (and singletons) in whom language is so disordered that there are long-term effects on behaviour and education. An example is a pair of boys who were just about to start school when they were brought to the paediatric clinic, scarcely able to say a word. It is clearly better not to wait until things reach that stage.

The earlier steps are taken, the better. Twins do best – and the outlook for their reading and behaviour also improves – if their language problems are dealt with by the age of four, and preferably by the age of three.

Although multiples may be prone to language problems, it is vital that causes are not missed. Since speech is learnt by imitating others, normal hearing is essential. As a family doctor, I would recommend a hearing test as a first step to take for any child (twin or singleton) who has any delay or abnormality in talking. Your health visitor or GP can arrange this. Hearing loss is more likely in a child who has had recurrent ear infections, but every so often a youngster who has never had earache has a substantial hearing deficit.

Assuming that your children's hearing is normal and that nobody suspects a communication disorder like autism, what should you do next?

If your twins are very young and the language problem is mild – say they are only a couple of months behind the expected stage in producing speech sounds – all that may be needed is individual attention. Reading to each separately on a daily basis, with his twin being entertained or supervised in another room, is one excellent way of doing this.

Since about 5 per cent of children have some language delay and most children recover from it, there is some debate as to what else should or can be done. With anything more than the mildest delay, it seems wise to see a speech therapist and get an opinion as to whether your child needs therapy. If possible, it may be worth getting a therapist who has experience of working with twins.

Your GP can refer you for speech therapy. You may have to wait some time for an appointment for an assessment, so don't delay setting the process in motion. While you are waiting, you can start reading to your children separately (if you don't already do this).

Identical twins tend to have similar language skills. All the same, it is not unknown for only one twin to need speech therapy, in which case one may gloat while the other is upset – and it is sometimes the one who is having therapy who acts superior! This situation needs tactful handling. There are no easy answers, and you will need to:

- ensure that neither twin thinks he is now 'better' than his sibling
- help the twin being treated and reinforce what he's learning
- prevent his 'untreated' sibling from persuading him to revert to his old speech errors.

· *The Secret Language of Twins* ·

I have already mentioned that twins communicate with each other, but how often do they use a private language that only they understand?

The secret language of twins (also known as idioglossia, cryptophasia or cryptoglossia) has been a subject of intense fascination for many years. It is quite true that a few twins may speak nothing but their 'own' language and every so often dramatic examples receive publicity.

Some researchers have suggested that, in toddlerhood, up

to 40 per cent of twins speak a secret language that nobody else, not even their parents, can understand, and that the proportion may be even higher in identical twins. This sensational figure may actually represent an illusion of a secret language, according to Professor Hay and a number of other experts. The private language can often be understood by outsiders who try hard. Research also shows that:

• young twins are good at understanding each other's speech and body language
• they make similar mistakes in speech
• because they tend to reinforce each other's mistakes, errors persist longer
• their language development can be delayed.

All in all, this is probably enough to give the impression that secret languages are common. If one listens carefully to a piece of so-called cryptoglossia, in many cases it's simply very immature speech.

What if your twins really do share their own language? The answer is that it doesn't matter provided that normal language is also developing at the right time. Come to think of it, many of us, for instance husbands and wives, use our own private words for things. As long as we can and do communicate normally with others, this is not important.

· *More than One Language* ·

Now that so much of our society is multicultural, there are many families where youngsters speak one language with their parents and another with their grandparents, childminder or at the nursery. Parents of children with speech delay often believe that the problem is due to learning more than one language at the same time.

A bilingual or even multilingual upbringing can certainly be confusing. For a while, young bilingual children tend to speak several languages in the same conversation or sentence, but the important point is that they speak as fluently as any child.

A bilingual upbringing is most unlikely to account for language delay. If one looks closely at many of the youngsters who don't speak, they are not actually speaking much in any language. The message is that if you think your twins have a language difficulty, get a proper assessment (including a hearing check), however many languages they are exposed to.

Chapter Ten

PRE-SCHOOL TWINS

The pre-school years cover the ages of about three to five years. It is a delightful time that many parents say brings the best of both worlds. Children are still very close to their mothers at this age, and most also get the chance of going to playgroup or nursery school for as many as twenty hours a week which brings opportunities for new experiences.

Although there are many advantages in the pre-school years – not least the fact that your youngsters are gradually growing up and becoming more biddable – there are several points to bear in mind:

- However good the local pre-school facilities are, parents – in practice, mothers – continue to be the main educators of children at this age.

- Pre-school twins still need a lot of adult time and attention – again, this probably means yours. That's something which is still in short supply, particularly if you are thinking of returning to work.

- The pre-school years are when many twins begin to be aware of their twinship and therefore of being different from most other children, who are singletons. This is at least partly because adults and other children perceive and treat them as unusual.

- This can result in twins being lumped together, which often marks the beginning of a lifelong battle to be valued for themselves.

I was so disappointed that, after three years of doing our best to help the children develop individuality, our efforts were completely undermined by a couple of mornings at playgroup. The leader obviously treated them as one and by the end of their second session the children were calling them 'Twins' instead of using their names.

• Unfortunately, many playgroups and nurseries are still inexperienced in the issues concerning multiple-birth children, even when they think they're not. You may have to be extra vigilant to make sure your children get the best out of any pre-school they attend.

    Multiples should be prioritized for pre-school and nursery education, but the level of provision varies around the country. There is a huge patchwork of public and private provision which affects what your family can be offered.

• The more you make of the pre-school years, the better prepared your children will be for their school career and the better they will probably do in both language and behaviour.

· *Pre-school Education* ·

Obviously, playgroups and nurseries give children the chance to get out of the house and away from their parents (unless they happen to be playgroup leaders). If nothing else, this helps to teach youngsters about separation, which is an important experience for many children, especially if they have never been looked after by a child-minder, nanny, or anyone else for any length of time.

Pre-school also gives young children exposure to a slightly more structured environment, which is good preparation for 'big school'.

Pre-school allows children to play with toys they don't

have at home and to experiment with a variety of new materials. For twins and other multiples, it provides vital opportunities for messy play, such as finger-painting, which they may not get in their own homes because the chaos would be unacceptable in the relatively civilized surroundings of the home. It also reinforces the enjoyment of singing, saying rhymes, listening to stories and looking at books, all of which are important in developing language and learning to read. This is the time when a young child's literacy and a love of books, as well as basic skills in writing and number, are established.

Play is actually a serious business, as educationalists emphasize. Take role play as an example. As well as being fun for all concerned, dressing up and taking on different roles enables a child to experience different situations and experiment with them. Through all kinds of play, a child learns about his environment. Headteacher Pat Preedy, who is also TAMBA's education research consultant, points out: 'Remember, play is not something that is given as a reward after work. Through play, the child builds firm foundations for later learning. Children who have difficulties with learning have often had impoverished play experiences.' She also adds that it is important for a child to learn sustained play, instead of flitting from one activity to another. This is something a number of twins are prone to do, perhaps because they are used to being distracted and interrupted.

The way a child tackles tasks is important too. Discussing an activity beforehand and afterwards is vital to taking the learning forward. The child who learns to 'play, do and review' acquires the ability to focus and stay on track, clearly a valuable life-skill.

Playgroups and nurseries also teach children elementary social skills, such as taking turns, something multiples especially need to acquire. Children aged three or more are usually ready to make friends outside the family and pre-school play provides good opportunities for mixing and playing alongside another child (other than the twin). However, for many multiples and their parents there can be practical problems which means that socializing comes less easily than it does to singletons.

· *Which Pre-school?* ·

Provision varies from area to area. At one extreme there may only be the chance of one or two two-hour sessions a week for your children at a playgroup in a local church hall, while at the other end of the spectrum there may be enough nursery places, attached to primary schools, for all children of pre-school age.

Most suburban areas fall somewhere in the middle, with many playgroups (which you have to pay for) offering a variety of hours and perhaps two or more State-run nursery schools with a long list of children waiting for spaces for sessions. These are usually held every morning (or afternoon) of the week, each session lasting two and a half hours.

In some areas, all pre-school children eventually get a nursery place, but perhaps only for one term just before they start primary school – equitable maybe, but of limited use. In Britain the new pre-school voucher scheme may give parents greater choice or it may not. It is a controversial issue and its impact is not yet known. The voucher scheme is however unlikely to increase the total number of places at either play-groups or nurseries.

You may be able to get your twins or triplets into a nursery school a term or two ahead of most singletons if you can convince the authorities that they have special needs. For example, you might emphasize the greater need they have to acquire social skills, or you could point out any learning or language difficulties they may already have. Gifted children too may qualify for early entry to nursery and possibly primary school. A developmental assessment (ask your family doctor how to get this) could help back up your request and you can also ask TAMBA for assistance. Unfortunately, showing that your children desperately need nursery places does not mean they will get them: there are often simply not enough places and the more multiples you have the greater the problem will be.

Faced with several possibilities for pre-school, look around at what is available nearby. Other things being equal, it ought to be nearby, not only to make it easy for you, but to enable your children to see their friends socially outside the playgroup, at birthday parties and so on.

Start your search early – no later than their second birthday and possibly much earlier – even if they cannot start until they are nearly three years old. Because you have more than one child, you have more decisions to make. You need more places too, so get their names down in plenty of time. It is not much good discovering that the ideal playgroup can accommodate only one of your triplets.

Don't be embarrassed about visiting lots of playgroups. You may need to in order to get a feel for what is on offer. You will have obvious questions about the cost and the number and length of sessions available (is each one long enough for you to get to the supermarket and back, for instance?). But you also need to ask a few searching questions, such as:

1   How structured are the sessions? Are children allowed to get on with their choice of activity or are they shepherded at predetermined times from one thing to the next? Is there any progression? For instance, are the older children (rising-fives) treated separately for part of the session, in preparation for school? If so, are twins automatically in the same group? This may be fine for

many multiples, but you have to decide what will be best for yours.

2   How is discipline achieved? Is it based just on verbal warnings, or is any exclusion or 'time out' meted out as punishment?

3   Does the playgroup leader or nursery teacher have any experience of multiples? Probably not, but this is a good opening question for introducing the subject. Perhaps the teacher has taught very few multiples, but has had literature from TAMBA or is planning to attend a course or study day. Experience is vital, but the right attitude is more important. Watch out for sweeping statements such as 'All twins are like that.' In reality, there are very few areas in which all twins are alike.

4   Check out the parents' rota – almost all playgroups have one, while nurseries don't normally count on parental help. Is a mother of triplets expected to help out three times as often? Clearly, you may have three times the usual number of children, but there's still only one of you and you should not be roped into doing a lot more than other parents.

5   If you are going to send both (or all) of your children to the same playgroup, ask about a bulk discount on fees. It sounds cheeky and you usually won't get one, but it does no harm to ask.

6   Don't forget to ask yourself whether you like the atmosphere of the playgroup. This may prove to be more important to you and your children than some of the other factors.

· *Together or Apart?* ·

Playgroup could give you an ideal opportunity to spend a little regular protected time with each child on her own, so should you send your twins together or not? This may be the first occasion you have to consider the question of separation, but it's an issue that will crop up again and again during your children's school careers.

It is impossible to say which option is better for twins in the long term. The research just has not been done and in any case the best course of action depends on your family. Your decision will be influenced by what is available, as well as by your own situation and preferences. Twins who show a little language delay or behaviour problems may benefit from separate playgroups, for instance, but if they have never been separated they are likely to find this traumatic.

Sometimes only one twin is ready for playgroup, just as one may be out of nappies before the other. It is usually right to send that child on ahead. Holding her back could be wrong – a good example of equal treatment being unfair. Besides, this may encourage her brother to become dry very soon.

If you have triplets or more, your options as well as your time will be more limited, but with twins there will usually be a little leeway. Here are some of the options:

1 You could send your children to the same playgroup on different days. In this way they will both benefit from similar experiences and learn about separation not only from you but from each other. By attending on different days, your twins are also less likely to be mistaken for each other – in theory, anyway! On the other hand, this gives you little or no time on your own and the child who is at home on a particular day may feel very left out unless you make an effort to do something with him.

For nearly half a term, James went on Mondays and Wednesdays, while Ben went on Tuesdays and Thursdays. Whoever was at home with me moped around and didn't really settle to anything, while I got increasingly harassed. It was my health visitor who pointed out that I was making a rod for my own back.

2 They could attend separate playgroups altogether. This will give you more time to yourself and they can benefit from the maximum number of sessions available. If they are ready and happy to be apart, this will work well, but if not they could view this enforced separation as a punishment or ordeal. You do need to consider the logistics as well. Ferrying them to different destinations can be hard, especially if you have other children too.

3 You could send them together. The children learn about separation from you without the trauma of breaking away from each other. You have to watch how the playgroup staff and helpers treat your twins. You may find them being constantly compared, confused or treated as a single unit. Other young children are often very good at knowing who is who, even with identicals, but if grown-ups constantly refer to your children as 'the twins' it will rub off.

I felt I could tell off the leader gently but it was a losing battle when all the other kids talked about 'the twins'. Even though they always knew which was which, it was as if they couldn't be bothered, and that wasn't healthy, in my opinion.

4 A solution that works very well for some parents is sending twins separately for one or two sessions a week, and together the rest of the time. However, this option leaves you having to entertain the one who is not at playgroup. Bear in mind that it also gives playgroup

leaders occasional scope for confusion; for example, 'You did a lovely picture yesterday, Harry. Or was that Jack?'

5   With nursery school there are fewer options, though you may be able to send one twin to morning sessions and the other in the afternoon. Timing during the lunch period can be a little tight, but this arrangement works well for some.

My mother had the girls separately. She'd have one in the morning and the other in the afternoon, which was nice for them and for her. In fact, she could really only manage one of my daughters at a time so it was an ideal arrangement for all concerned, provided I came back from work at lunchtime and gave her a hand.

· *When Your Children are at* ·
Pre-school

As a parent, there are many things you can do to help your twins or triplets get the most from playgroup or nursery:

● Twins shouldn't have to do everything together. Co-operation may make some things happen, but it can also hinder learning and the development of their individuality. They also need to learn the skill of co-operating with other children, not just each other.

   So if your children aren't already placed in separate groups within the nursery, ask if they could be. Some teachers put them together 'to help them settle in', then forget all about separating them later. In reality, few twins need to sit side by side the whole time – even pairs who are very dependent on each other are usually happy as long as each knows where the other is.

- Help the staff and other parents to distinguish between your children, though preferably not with labels or with jumpers emblazoned with their names. Names on the front of a young child's clothing (or, for that matter, on her gym bag, lunch box, etc.) can be a distinct disadvantage and even a security hazard, since any stranger will know what she's called. Far better to use different clothing (hairstyles too if you can) so that playgroup and nursery staff can tell your twins apart at a glance.

- When do other children treat twins as a single unit? Only when adults have taught them to. You can at least ensure that *you* always refer to them by name.

  I knew I'd won when one of the other mothers on the parents' rota spent two mornings helping before she even realized Alex and Kim were related. The fact that they were each dressed very differently certainly helped.

- Dress them for mess: they will be absolutely filthy by the end of the morning and you may go berserk if they are covered in flour and face paint when you pick them up. If they wear clothes that don't matter, you will feel a lot better about it. Wet wipes kept in the car will help deal with sticky hands and, incidentally, a couple of plastic carrier bags in the boot to transport still-wet works of art are also a good idea.

- When you pick them up, ask each child separately about how the day went. Twins rarely have any privacy and it is something they often guard jealously. Your children also need to know you are interested in them as individuals. So don't let one of them spill the beans to you about his twin's news, no matter how keen he is.

- Similarly, if you want to know if Becky cried when you left, or was banished to the corner for any misdemeanours, it is best to ask an adult rather than her brother Sam.

Besides, you may get a pack of lies: many of them seem to enjoy getting their twin into trouble and will go to some lengths to do so.

- Try to appreciate their efforts, be they lopsided fairy cakes, loo-roll sculptures or pictures made of pasta shapes. It is important to make the right noises, even though you will have twice as many of these to take home as the other mothers and the novelty will undoubtedly wear off before long.

- If your twins are very different in ability or interests, try to avoid negative comparisons. One child's painting may look absolutely pathetic next to his twin's competent self-portrait, but with a little thought one can always find something to say that's positive, amusing or even important-sounding. One mother opted for: 'That's a great style, Gregory – I think it might even be cubist.'

- When it is your turn to help out, keep in the background, but take the opportunity to watch your children during the session. You may be surprised by how differently they behave at playgroup. On the other hand, it may be just like it is at home. One mother of triplets commented that at playgroup hers just functioned as a pack for months, roaming together with hardly any interaction with other children. This can also be true of quads and more.

- When they start making friends, be prepared for plenty of cries of "'s not fair!' One of your children may well be invited out more than his twin, at least to begin with. When one is asked round to tea at a friend's, don't be tempted to ask if his twin can come too. Instead, try to make that time more interesting for the one who has not been invited. Do something nice, just the two of you. Go swimming, perhaps, since that's hard with two children. Or else ask another little friend round to your place for him to play with while his twin is out. Eventually he'll be asked out too, and the score usually evens up. It doesn't always, but then life is unfair.

· *Preparing for 'Big School'* ·

Whether your children are at playgroup or nursery school, or at home with you, the pre-school years are vital in terms of preparing them for primary school and the rest of their scholastic career. In general, the more you do to promote your twins' individualities and identities now at this stage, the easier their schooldays will be – though not always! It is surprising how many twins still share not just a bedroom but a bed at the age of four or five.

- Don't go in for techniques such as cramming, rote learning or other methods to speed up learning. These are not so much learning methods as party pieces and, however impressed other mothers may be, you will probably not be helping your children at all.

- Encourage each child to learn to concentrate, whether it is on a book, a jigsaw or a construction toy, for five to ten minutes at a time despite the presence of his twin. This is desperately difficult for many twins to learn because they are so used to interfering with each other's activities.

- Teach them to take turns. This is another skill that's vital for success in the classroom and the playground, one you can teach quite simply with almost any daily activities.

- Help them communicate. As mentioned in the previous chapter, twins often excel at interrupting. Many of them need to be taught to speak at an appropriate pace.

- Encourage your children to talk without shouting. I know this is difficult in a household full of noisy youngsters, and you are likely to be shouting much of the time too, if only to make yourself heard above the din, but it is worth a try.

- Extend their vocabulary and language skills as best you can. This means talking to each child clearly, slowly enough and appropriately (with actions that match what you are saying to that child). Remember to make eye contact with the one you are addressing.

- Make looking at books fun. Borrow a variety of books from the library. Your youngsters can have their own tickets from an early age (incidentally, there are often no fines payable on children's tickets) and will enjoy 'turning them into books' at the borrowing desk. Talk about the books you liked or have enjoyed, and read to them. It is still helpful to read to each twin separately if you can, but a bedtime story read together is better than none at all.

- Set a good example: households where adults enjoy reading tend to nurture youngsters who do too. Encourage your twins to talk and think about things. You could ask questions such as 'Why do you think that bus is going so slowly now that it is raining?' If you don't know the answer to something they ask, resolve (at least occasionally) to look it up and let them know what it is. It will be ages before they are able to use encyclopaedias or dictionaries themselves, but that's not the point – the aim is to encourage enquiring minds and show that the answers can be found if one looks.

- Teach your children how to dress themselves. This applies to singletons too, though with twins it is even more tempting (and a lot faster) to dress them yourself, but they need to learn to do it themselves. Watch out for twins who dress each other: in a boy–girl pair, the girl will sometimes dress her brother.

- Let each have a little privacy from his twin whenever possible. Most twins share a bedroom at this age, but they needn't always both play in it at the same time. Increase one-to-one contact if you can, with separate outings, for example.

- As in earlier years, avoid labelling or creating artificial distinctions between them.

- Treat your child in a way that is appropriate for his age. Your twins are growing up. Of course, the children are growing all the time, but it is often hard for a parent to notice it, especially when their pre-school children are still in a buggy, or are very cute, as is often the case with multiples.

- Be positive about school. If you didn't enjoy your own schooldays, either keep quiet about it, or be selective about what you say. 'I didn't like my school-bag because it was brown' is less alarming than the fact that you were scared stiff of the headteacher. In fact, be positive about the future generally if you can.

Finally, prepare yourself for the time when your children will go off to school for several hours every day, leaving you, perhaps for the first time since their birth, with the luxury of deciding what *you* want to do – whether it is returning to work with a merchant bank or learning to arrange flowers. Faced with the all-consuming demands of rearing twins or more, you may have lost touch with some of the things that mattered to you. If you have, the start of term in September may be something of a milestone, giving you the chance to spend a little thought on yourself. Far be it from me to suggest that the most important benefit to you will be more free time. One of the most exciting aspects of having twins start school is seeing them enjoy new experiences, and sharing these enthusiastically with you.

My daughters greeted me outside the classroom, their cheeks glowing and their eyes like saucers. They were burning to tell me their latest discovery – that they like fish-fingers.

Your life may also feel a little empty when your 'babies' begin at primary school. Strangely enough, it is sometimes the mothers who have always had their own careers who feel most bereft when their twins start school.

Chapter Eleven

PRIMARY SCHOOL

The best years of their lives? Perhaps: primary school is an exciting time, full of opportunities for making friends and learning new skills, before the demands of homework, tests and exams become all-consuming. But there can be problems and every year TAMBA receives an increasing number of requests for help with twins at primary school and beyond.

Parents occasionally have concerns about their twins' education because of earlier problems with prematurity or growth retardation, or perhaps because one of them spent time in special care as a baby. Past medical or physical disorders can sometimes affect a youngster's school career. Even when they don't, it can be hard to trust that all will be well for your children at school when they had such an uncertain start in life. Understandably, some parents continue to have anxieties about their once sickly offspring for many years.

How will your twins fare? Several research projects have focused on the performance of twins and more at primary school. The first large-scale observations came from Australia, from a nationwide study which began in 1985 and also from the La Trobe University Twin Study which, starting in 1978, looked at how twins progressed in terms of behaviour and skills both at home and at school.

Now new studies have shed valuable light on how twins do at primary school in the UK. Pat Preedy, a headteacher at Knowle Infant School in the Midlands, began her research into twins at school when, in 1992, she found a record nine sets of twins in her nursery and reception classes. Spurred on by TAMBA, she has now carried out a national survey of 2993 schools and how they deal with multiples, covering 11 878 twins, 351 triplets and five sets of quins in all. Later in this chapter we shall examine some of Pat Preedy's findings (and those of others) which are relevant to parents.

· *Together or Apart?* ·

Whether or not twins should be put in the same class at school or apart is not necessarily the most crucial issue where their education is concerned, but it has huge practical implications and must be considered early on. Most parents have some choice in the matter, though circumstances may dictate what you do if, for instance:

- one of your twins has special needs
- you have a boy–girl pair and you intend to educate them in the independent sector (where schools are still often segregated by sex even at the pre-prep stage)
- you live in a small rural community.

As one parent says:

> Before we moved here, we were told it was county policy to split twins up and put them in separate classes within a school, but when we investigated we found that all three local primary schools had only one intake. Separating our two girls would have involved different schools, with all the attendant problems of that, and we couldn't have coped.

A word about 'policy' later, but first let's look at the potential advantages and drawbacks of separating twins at primary level.

Twins who are in the same class may:

- derive so much benefit from each other's support that it is easier for them to be separated from their home and parents

- benefit academically from competing against each other (when they are very similar in ability, each acts as a pacemaker for the other)

- be very confusing for teachers, especially if identical – but some teachers also fail to distinguish between non-identicals of the same sex

- distract each other, to the detriment of their learning and behaviour (this tends to happen most when they are sitting next to, or close to, each other)

- constantly check up on each other's work (and cramp their twin's style)

- function only as a unit, with one child taking on certain tasks and his twin the others

- co-operate so closely that they copy each other's work, either in class or at home

- be suspected of cheating, even when they don't collaborate; after all, many twins simply make the same mistakes

- try to get each other into trouble, with one twin accusing the other of misdemeanours he committed himself

- collude in or cover up any misbehaviour so that adults don't know whom to blame or punish

- try to attract attention in class by behaving badly

- present problems if they are of different ability and one constantly lags behind

- create difficulties when one is dominant and the other so dependent on him that he appears unable to work or socialize on his own

- be unfairly compared – even when they are so similar in ability that they resemble each other more closely than they resemble any other child in the class, some teachers and parents will draw unflattering and unhelpful comparisons between twins.

Twins in separate classes may:

- make their own friends more easily (but this is not always so – remember that primary school lasts only six hours a day and some of that time is spent in the playground)

- be less confusing for teachers; the staff may also get to know each twin better

- be able to progress at their own pace without worrying about their twin's performance – this is important when they are very different in ability or attitude

- enjoy more privacy, something that twins rarely have

- behave better in class because of lack of distraction from their twin

- compete less and therefore behave better

- have more stimulating or interesting things to say to each other at the end of the day

- compare their teachers – and find one of them lacking! (This last factor can become an issue if teaching or discipline styles are very different. For instance, one twin may consistently get higher marks or more house points when both his work and his behaviour were no different from his sister's.)

So, together or apart? No single answer is right for every family and it is a question of which is more likely to bring out the best in your twins. Most educationalists would agree that there is no evidence that separate classes *per se* really aid the individual development of twins. In deciding what suits your children, you will have to take two main factors into account: the twins' relative abilities and their relationship with each other.

If you have a boy–girl pair, teachers will have few problems telling them apart, but a potential difficulty is that girls are often more advanced, especially in language, and may take charge in class (she may do her twin's work for him too).

If one twin is dominant, the dependent one may benefit from being in a separate class (or even a different school), though the dominant one may find it hard being on his own to begin with.

Do your twins function well independently? If so, separation is less of an issue, but if one tends to opt out of activities, they may both benefit from being apart.

Are there obvious physical differences between them? A twin who is less confident because he is shorter, less healthy or less co-ordinated than his brother may improve in self-esteem once out of his twin's shadow.

Consider how competitive they are. Does each concentrate well or are they distracted by each other? Sometimes like-minded twins can be a combustible mixture.

What else is going on in the family – a divorce, bereavement or house move? At such difficult times, twins can derive a lot of comfort from being together, so perhaps a separation can be postponed.

Many twins starting school have rarely been apart, as Pat Preedy's work confirms. Some pairs may have been separated only when some unpleasant incident has occurred, for instance when one of them has had to go into hospital. Under these circumstances both will need extra support and understanding at school.

Have your twins been away from home already, for instance at nursery? How often and for how long are they normally apart? Perhaps they spend weekends with grandparents separately. Think about their perceptions of being apart; is it fun, or a punishment to be endured? Do they like each other's company? It is worth considering all these points. You won't necessarily do something just because the youngsters suggest it, but their views ought to be taken into account. Twinship creates a special bond which one should neither ignore nor try to break forcibly.

Triplets and more

If you decide to separate your triplets into different classes, how can this be achieved? A few schools may have three parallel classes, which makes it feasible, but most don't because they are just not big enough. Putting the closer pair together in one class can work, although the third one may feel left out on her own. For some triplet families, a reasonable solution is to separate the one who is of different gender; another is to put the non-identical pair together. You may be happy for them to be at two or more different schools, but bear in mind the extra effort involved, especially if they have different term-times.

> Actually I enjoyed having the kids at home at different times
> in half-terms and holidays. It didn't happen often, but when
> it did it meant special days with just one or two of my
> triplets instead of the whole trio.

On the other hand, there's no reason why placing all your triplets (or quads) in the same class will not work, especially if they are in different groups within the class. It is just that the more children you have, the fewer your options. A school may even refuse to give you places for all three 'on principle': it has been known for headteachers to believe they cannot possibly make that many places available to just one family. Remember that you have the right to appeal against decisions you believe are not in your children's best interests.

School policies

Some schools or education departments have a policy on twins, usually to separate them in two classes (or, less often, to place them together) regardless of the circumstances.

It can only be wrong to have a fixed strategy for dealing with twins and higher multiples. As educationalists with a special interest in multiples sometimes say, the best policy is no policy – or, rather, no rigid policy. Twins have to be educated on their own merits and a blanket ruling may just be a cover for not thinking properly about the issues.

If the school's prevailing policy happens to fit in with what you wanted for your children anyway, that's fine. If not, you can question it. TAMBA can advise parents on this and may be able to write a letter to support your point of view.

In practice

What happens where there is no firm policy on multiples? The decision as to how to place them is usually made collectively by headteachers, class teachers and parents. If your opinion is not sought, ensure you make it known. Sometimes a decision is made to keep twins and more together on somewhat arbitrary grounds, for instance date of birth!

In practice, most twins start primary school in the same class. Preedy's research showed that twice as many children were together as were apart at primary level. Many twins are happy to start school if they know they won't be separated. In this way they can learn to become independent of you without having to be apart from each other at the same time. This makes a few mothers feel left out:

> On the first day, they went off together into the classroom without so much as a backward glance, while I stood there with a great big lump in my throat.

If your twins are in the same class, it is usually best for them to be placed in separate groups within the class to avoid being lumped together, distracting each other or collaborating when they should be working independently.

Sam and Robert were seated side by side in their new school, but they never settled because they were constantly fighting instead of getting on with it. The teacher called me in to say she was having terrible trouble with my boys and what did I think was the matter – was there a problem at home? And I had to explain to her that it was really her doing. They were no trouble at all when they were placed at separate tables and in fact soon outperformed all the other children in the class! I was bursting with pride when I realized what they were capable of achieving.

Many twins end up in different classes later in their primary school careers, with a decision to separate them being taken at the end of the reception year, or later. Some pairs go their separate ways at the age of seven. Take care, whenever they separate, however: if one child stays with his original class and the other goes to a different one, leaving his friends as well as his twin could be a big wrench for him. He may, understandably, resent this and find it an uphill struggle to start all over again with a new group, while his twin has no problems.

When they are placed in different classes, it can be helpful for each to see the other one's classroom, so that he can picture where his twin will spend most of the day. If they are at different schools, this can be even more important.

Taking stock

No decision you make should be truly irreversible: you don't always know at the time what is right and parenting as a whole is a huge experiment. It is a good idea to reappraise progress every so often, possibly at the end of the school year or whenever you or the teachers think it advisable. The important thing is to be flexible. It doesn't really matter whether your children are together or apart, as long as they are happy and making good progress. And that depends a lot on the attitudes towards them at school and at home.

· *Teachers and Twins* ·

Thanks to the efforts of TAMBA, MBF and the families of twins themselves, there is increasing awareness of the issues of multiples at school, but even so some professionals remain unenlightened. Almost every teacher in the UK is likely to come across at least one set of twins in his or her career, yet formal training for teachers does not cover this area.

Some teachers therefore have little choice but to generalize from the previous set of twins they taught, but of course there is no such thing as 'typical twins'. A few twins are hardly aware of each other, while others are intimately inter-reliant and others still fight non-stop in class (not yours, you hope . . .).

At the start of the school year, you may not know what your children's teachers' experiences of multiples are. The chances are that the staff will all want to do their best for your twins and that they will be open-minded. I have certainly found this, and my own twins have had some teachers of the highest calibre. However, I think it's realistic not to take for granted that your children's teachers are well-versed in handling multiples. For instance, one or two parents have discovered that their twins have had just one combined baseline assessment between them. Such situations could perhaps be avoided by trying to find out early in the school year how a teacher handles twins in class.

Unfortunately a lot of classroom material is unhelpful. Twins are popular in print and reading schemes are no exception. They are often full of stories about highly stereotypical twins – the kind whom nobody can distinguish, who always speak simultaneously, dress in identical clothes and want to do the same things side by side 'because they are twins'.

Many teachers are eager and willing to know more, and we are all learning constantly. Everyone involved, whether parents or teachers, should be humble enough at least to listen to one another. In your dealings with your twins' teachers, co-operation rather than confrontation is the best strategy. Keep lines of communication open by meeting often. This will also ensure that you are aware of what is going on in class.

Your children's school may like to know about the educational opportunities provided by TAMBA and MBF. TAMBA also publishes an excellent general leaflet for schools; every school should have a copy.

There is a great deal schools could do to help multiples if only staff were aware of the issues. Together with TAMBA, Pat Preedy has drafted a framework policy to enable schools to best consider the needs of twins and higher-order births (see the Appendix, page 339).

· *How Multiples Do at School* ·

Most twins go through school without any major problems, but (as with any children) they occasionally have difficulties, especially with language and reading. Are these any more common in twins?

There are no consistent differences between singletons and multiples in intelligence, or in Maths and other subjects, but Australian research strongly suggests that reading problems are more common in twins, especially boys. While the Australian work shows that most twins have no problems, it highlights the suspicion that difficulties at school are more likely in:

* identical (MZ) twins
* male twins
* those with a sibling only two to three years older
* those who speak a language other than English at home.

It would not be too controversial to add birth complications and other medical problems to this list of risk factors.

There is some controversy about how twins perform at school and new evidence from the UK indicates that they do no worse than singletons. so twinning in itself does not seem to be a handicap in terms of achievement.

The recent PIPS (Performance Indicators in Primary Schools) Project has focused on the progress children make in school. It was set up to look at the value added by education, so to speak: it is well known, for instance, that some schools have better results, but in some cases this is because they select more able or more privileged pupils. In other words, to know how well a school does, one has to consider the level at which each child started at, and then assess the child's progress relative to that. The PIPS project compared children at the same starting point and looked at where they were expected to finish. If children achieve more than expected, then this is the value added.

The PIPS project doesn't study only twins, but it has identified the twins and multiples within a large sample of children. Peter Tymms of Durham University and Pat Preedy have looked at the scores of multiples and so far the results are encouraging. Their data show that twins and other multiples:

- don't seem to be disadvantaged compared with singletons when they start primary school
- probably do just as well as singletons in their first year at school
- don't differ appreciably from singletons in 'early literacy' scores (pre-reading skills).

These results seem to conflict with those of the earlier Australian work. Which are right? Possibly both. The studies looked at different populations at different times, so there could be cultural differences, for a start. In 1990s Britain there may also be greater awareness of twins' issues. It could also be relevant that the recent increase in multiple births is largely amongst women over 35, who are often more advantaged and educated to a higher level than younger mothers.

Thus far, PIPS has analysed the first couple of years at school. Differences may emerge later in twins' school careers.

One reassuring finding from the British research is that multiples are good at early language skills. One possible explanation is that, whatever happens subsequently, twins and higher-order multiples probably have the same potential for language and reading as singletons. Therefore, it is then up to parents and teachers to help them fulfil that potential.

· *Possible Problems at School* ·

Problems tend to crop up with twins from time to time. It's tempting to assume that they will grow out of their difficulty, or that it has happened simply because they are twins. Occasionally both are true, but sometimes action can and should be taken.

Reading

Many children have trouble reading. Some learn later than others, some read inaccurately and a few seem competent but just don't enjoy it much. Nevertheless, the Australian survey suggests that twin boys with reading difficulty differ in some ways from singletons who don't read well:

- they are more likely to have speech problems
- they may also spell poorly
- they tend to read the letter b for d (and vice versa)
- they read quickly but inaccurately, as if they are rushing it
- they sometimes have trouble with numbers too.

Reading difficulties may improve in time, but they don't always. If one of your twins seems to have trouble, it is worth doing something about it early on in his school career, as so much depends on being able to read well. You will need to liaise closely with the teacher and may also need the advice of an educational psychologist. It is also worth checking your child's eyesight.

Needs vary from child to child. Sometimes all that's required is help from a parent with reading at home. If you do this, make sure that your child learns to read accurately. Don't just move your finger under the text: twins tend to rush and may not understand, so take it slowly and ask your child questions to check his comprehension.

Learning support is sometimes necessary. This usually takes place at school, but, wherever reading problems are dealt with, you need to co-operate closely with the teacher. There is more about special educational needs in Chapter 14.

If only one of your children is poor at reading, help him accept this with equanimity. It is hard to be different from (especially less good than) your twin when the whole world expects you to be just the same. Teach him to see that no two people are the same at everything, whether it is football or reading. But don't ignore the achievements of the more able twin!

Bad behaviour

Problems are by no means inevitable, but of these bad behaviour is probably the biggest issue at school as well as at home. It may be linked with language and reading problems, but this isn't always the case. In fact, very able children often misbehave most because they are bored and also because their intellectual abilities outstrip their social skills. According to teachers and parents of twins, certain styles of behaviour seem to cause upheaval most often. These are discussed below.

Fighting and aggressive behaviour

Fighting, covered in Chapter 9, is certainly more common in twins, especially boys of primary-school age.

> I thought everything was fine because they'd become so settled at home. But one of the other kids in their class informed me that they were always hitting each other at playtime. It was true, as I discovered from many subsequent meetings with their teacher. I actually began to dread seeing her outside the school at three-thirty and feared that she was scanning the horizon for me in order to lodge yet another complaint.

Often the children's aggression is seen only within the twinship: they may kick each other mercilessly at the slightest provocation, yet not lay a finger on other children.

One of the difficulties is trying to unravel what happened at school. This can be hard enough for a teacher to sort out even at the time of the incident. By the time your twins come out of school in the afternoon and give you their versions of events – often simultaneously and at full blast – the stories may have got garbled out of all recognition.

One cannot always know who started it or why, and often it doesn't much matter. The point is that children who fight have to learn that it gets them nowhere.

It can be hard to discipline twins, especially those who seem to have little need of adult approval. However, even singletons cannot be *forced* to do something, you can only make children *want* to do it.

On the whole, a school is best equipped to deal with school-based problems, but schools need full parental support. In handling twins who fight, it helps to:

- keep them constantly occupied
- help them make their own friends
- reward good behaviour

- ensure that fighting results in loss of privileges (don't relent when they hug you apologetically two minutes after the latest brawl).

A little distance between warring twins can also work wonders. This may be a good opportunity for more separate outings, or for considering separate bedrooms if you can arrange it. Often one twin is aggressive because he feels put upon, left behind or inferior in some way. If so, improving his self-esteem could dramatically reduce his tendency to outbursts of violence or angry frustration.

Competition

This may be another facet of the same problem – rivalry. It can also be, like fighting, an expression of a need for attention. Some competition is healthy: one twin may set standards that the other strives to achieve (and if he is of similar ability, he may well succeed).

> My two boys are like two peas in a pod in looks and academic work. In the same class they were thought to be a potential disaster because of fighting, but there was no choice at the local school, which only had one intake. However it worked out really well. They egg each other on so that they are both at the top of the class (jointly because their marks are identical). They are more than a year ahead in Maths and many other subjects. Their older sister is just as bright but doesn't often achieve as much. Being a singleton, perhaps she just doesn't have that competitive edge.

However, competition between twins can also lead to rushed work, mistakes, interrupting each other in class, finishing sentences for each other – and seriously getting on the teacher's nerves if the twins are in the same class.

They may also compete for friends and in sports. If they

are in different school houses, on sports day one may be elated while his twin is miserable.

> I knew they were each capable of good work, but they were so busy checking on each other's progress (and trying to finish first) even when they weren't in close proximity in class. I think they hardly ever achieved what they could have. If I placed the girls where they couldn't see each other, they'd still turn around and crane their necks . . . .

Some teachers comment on twins' constant awareness of each other's presence and movements both in class and outside it. If this becomes disruptive and wastes time in class it may be better to separate them into two different classes.

· *Comparisons between Twins* ·

We all compare things and people and when there is another child of exactly the same age the temptation is pretty well overwhelming for most people. On some levels it is useful: you may be able to tell that Natalie has a fever because her forehead feels so much hotter than Lorraine's, for example.

Most of the time it is less helpful. Strangely, one often compares twins' abilities when the differences between them are actually minute, which magnifies their importance out of all proportion. It is quite common for one twin to be regarded as less able, or even slow, when his performance is actually very like his twin's. He may even be well ahead of most of the class in that area, but the fact that his twin has a slight advantage over him can take on an unhealthy prominence in parents' minds – and often the children's too. It is not unknown for a difference of two percentage points in a Maths test to result in a punch-up.

Most parents cherish their twins' differences, which

makes it especially hard to avoid comparisons. But comparisons can seriously affect the children's own perceptions, expectations and ambitions, and could critically injure the confidence of one of them. Another danger is that, like labels, comparisons are sometimes wrong. For now, Ruth may be the better reader, but a few weeks later Becky might have taken off.

Different abilities

A more able child can easily outshine his twin's efforts. On the other hand, sometimes he may help him so effectively with schoolwork that differences in ability go unnoticed for some time.

It becomes very difficult for parents when there are real differences in ability or performance. If one child achieves more, the other necessarily achieves less. If one is a winner, the other is by definition the loser. We say we all love our children equally, and perhaps some of us do, but there is no doubt that some families – university lecturers' and musicians' families are two obvious examples – put a very high premium on certain talents and achievements and may discount others.

It is important to find something that the less academic child is good at, and to celebrate his achievements. Otherwise self-esteem can become seriously low. Sometimes twins can usefully be channelled into different activities, especially in a choice of sport or musical instrument, but one mustn't invent differences in interests or ignore the children's own preferences and talents. Perhaps they really do both want to learn the violin, play football or go to Brownies. It might, paradoxically, be better for their development as individuals to let them both do the same activities. But if you can manage it, it is sometimes beneficial for the children to do them separately from one other.

· *The joys* ·

Like most parenting books, this one concentrates on the hurdles and demands of bringing up children – in this case, multiples. But twins starting at primary school can bring great joy to their parents and it is worth pausing to enjoy the fun and count the advantages. Here are some parents' comments:

> I went back to work. Life was finally normal again.

> I was thrilled that we'd actually got to this stage. When they were tiny and premature there were days when it seemed impossible.

> The best thing? Without doubt it is the first school photo. Other parents just get a picture of one child, but I had one taken of them together, their faces scrubbed, their eyes shiny, their ties wonky as usual.

> They love school and have rushed off happily every morning almost without exception. But equally they're always thrilled to see me in the playground when they come out. Every afternoon I'm practically knocked over as they race to greet me with a double helping of hugs and cuddles. I know other mothers envy me too.

> They are making new friends. Twins seem popular with other children, and none of the kids has trouble telling them apart.

> Two lots of artwork to treasure. I even had some of their paintings framed. They look wonderful hanging side by side.

And before long no doubt you will find other benefits too.

· *What Parents Can Do* ·

- Help each child look and feel like an individual. This is especially important for single-sex pairs, but school uniforms don't help. Girls (and some boys) can have different hairstyles. It is often possible to customize school uniform for example:
  - pinafore for one, skirt for the other
  - different styles of jumper
  - different shades of grey trousers or skirts
  - different shoes, overcoats and school-bags.

In one school, one boy was allowed to wear the old-style school tie while his twin had the newer type. Different clothing is also an aid to safety.

- Don't refer to your children as 'the twins' or 'the triplets' if you can help it. If you need a collective noun, call them 'my/the children'.

- Be alert for teachers and anyone else who treats them as one unit. You can point out gently that this is unhelpful and even hurtful or unsettling for the children. One mother was most distressed to find the teacher referred to her two as Pinky and Perky, and soon, unfortunately, their classmates did the same.

- Encourage each child to take in his own notes or messages for the teacher, dinner money, etc., in separate envelopes. Otherwise some pairs may allot roles and insist that, for example, 'only Kim takes notes for the school office'.

- Ask your children every so often whether the teacher gets them mixed up. You might be surprised to hear that some twins get inaccurate educational assessments because staff cannot reliably tell them apart.

- Does one child usually tell you the other's news? Encourage each twin to talk to you in turn about her day at school. Ask, 'Danielle, how was your day?' Even if her verdict is 'Nothing' or "s boring', she should have a chance to get your full attention. They will eventually learn to take turns.

- Children need personal space in the literal sense too, but twins rarely get it. If they still share a bedroom, perhaps each could have his own desk or bookshelf.

- Help each child make his own friends. There may be difficulties to begin with, especially if neither has made many friends before, or one of them receives more invitations than the other.

- Make a special time to read each child's end-of-term report, if necessary using a kitchen timer to show them you're being scrupulously fair.

- Make sure you congratulate each child on his achievements. Some parents (and teachers) go out of their way not to congratulate a twin who has succeeded well at something, for fear of upsetting the other one. While it is true that the twin who has not done as well as his brother may take it badly, it makes no sense to punish, in effect, the one who comes first by withholding your praise. Like any child, he needs to have a bit of a fuss made over him. This can be quite a tightrope to tread, but would anything else be fair?

· *Dealings with Teachers* ·

- Don't assume that school life simply mirrors what happens at home. Sometimes twins fight at home but not at school, and vice versa. As one seven-year-old explained: 'I can't be good all the time.'

- Make yourself accessible to the teachers, ready to talk through any niggles as they arise, before they become major worries. Teachers appreciate this and you may well have a better relationship with them as a result.

- Always mention any medical problems or domestic difficulties which may affect your children's behaviour or performance at school.

- Don't forget to ask the teacher if she ever gets your children muddled (very important if they are in the same class). You might be surprised how often teachers confuse identicals – and even non-identicals of the same sex. There may be ways you can help her distinguish them.

- Find out what is happening in class. Are your children in separate groups, for instance? Does each approach the teacher for help? If so, is it for himself or for his sibling? Is each child treated on his own merits? You may be surprised to find out that some teachers will hold back one child (with spellings, times tables, reading or whatever) if his twin is not ready yet.

- What happens at playtime? Do your children just play together or do they mix well with others?

- Liaise with the teacher over sensible homework arrangements. You probably won't be able to help quite as much with your children's homework if you have twins – still less if you have triplets or quads. If each has to read to you in the evening, it makes more sense for your twins to have different books. Find out too about such things as project work. Your children may fight over who takes out which library book on Vikings, for instance. Make sure that your children aren't being given identical homework assignments simply because they are twins, while everyone else in the class does something different (this has been known to happen).

- On school outings, same-sex multiples probably ought to be in separate groups on grounds of safety if nothing else.

- Arrange separate appointments on parents' evenings for each child: perhaps some other parents could go in between your two appointments, just to keep the boundaries clear.

- Don't compare your children. Even for determined parents, this is surprisingly hard to avoid, but each child has to be considered – and encouraged – in his own right.

Treating multiples as individuals is as important at school as it is anywhere else, but of course they are still twins, no matter how different or alike they may be. For many people around them this in itself will be a source of interest, curiosity – and often intense satisfaction too. And why shouldn't one be allowed to enjoy the fact that twinship is special?

Chapter Twelve

SECONDARY SCHOOL

Whatever choices you made for your children's primary schooling, fresh decisions have to be made about their secondary education, and here a whole new set of circumstances need to be considered – all at the awkward time when your offspring are turning into teenagers.

As well as providing an education, secondary schools offer more of an opportunity for twins to become independent of each other, while still enjoying the pleasures that their special bond brings.

You could just send them both to the nearest secondary school and be done with it. After all, isn't that where everyone in your road goes? This may be the right decision in the end, but all the options – and there are now more of them – have to be explored first.

· *Same School* ·

The same school is the logical choice for many multiples, especially if they are of similar interests and abilities. Adolescents need personal space – and twins need it more than most – but secondary schools, which are often much bigger than primary schools, may provide it without your having to resort to difficult (and possibly divisive) arrangements involving different schools.

Same school, same class

There may simply be no choice, for instance if the school has only one class per year group, though this is unusual in a secondary school. Where there are two or more parallel classes, your twins may well end up in the same one if you don't ask, purely on the basis of their date of birth or the place of their surname in the alphabet!

Being in the same class is not usually the ideal option at secondary level. As at primary school, there could be intense competition between the children and unfair comparisons may be made. Adolescents tend to be even more touchy and in greater need of privacy than younger children, and often thrive better if they have space. This applies especially to those same-sex pairs where there are marked physical differences between them.

Nothing is ever totally black or white, however, and the same class may well work if your children function independently and are of similar ability. Bear in mind, though, that only one of them will be able to come top (or bottom, for that matter) and this can be a big issue at a sensitive age.

Same school, separate classes

Many secondary schools have parallel intakes and two or more classes all the way through. Moreover, your children's existing friends from primary school will probably be distributed more or less equally into the different classes, which could ease the separation of your twins from each other.

My identical boys started at the local comprehensive two years ago and we have no regrets so far. It is a huge school with plenty going on, and both Richard and Magnus have plenty of scope. They've made friends there – in fact, they each had people they knew from primary school in their class when they started. In their lunch break they each pursue activities. Richard does basketball and Magnus is into chess.

For many families, then, this will be the ideal time to put twins or triplets into separate classes. If your children are at an independent school, it may even precipitate a decision to transfer them to their next school at eleven plus rather than at thirteen plus, as many prep schools still do.

One family with gifted twin daughters transferred them from their small local primary school to a grammar school (grant-maintained) a year early. This enabled the girls finally to be in separate classes, ending years of intense and at times unhealthy rivalry between them. It is unusual to skip an academic year, but these girls found it easy and it worked well, not only because they were very able, but also because they were advanced physically.

Bear in mind, though, that even in separate classes your twins may still be taught together for some subjects and will probably mix in the playground, for sports and for some extra-curricular activities.

In some schools, pupils are streamed according to ability. It could lead to a strained situation if your twins or triplets then end up in different streams. A parent's sensitive handling can do a lot to help children come to terms with this, but do consider that it may be better for them to go to entirely different schools. There may also be problems if multiples of the same ability end up in the same set or stream.

· *Separate Schools* ·

TAMBA's secondary education advisor Rachel Hudson points out that this can work better than many parents imagine at first. Kids of secondary-school age often take themselves to school and enjoy both the freedom and responsibility this brings. Ferrying them to different addresses need not be a problem, depending on local transport and distance. Some evenings they may need chauffeuring, for instance if one or other has stayed late for an after-school activity.

Transport can prove expensive if one school is out of the immediate area. In these cases free or reduced fare travel may not be available. You will have to think about different sports days, different term-times and so on.

Incidentally, parents of singletons may gloomily inform you that different schools make uniforms an even more expensive proposition, but this is not really a consideration for families of multiples. Your children, being the same age, were unlikely ever to benefit from one handing on clothes to the other.

Separate schools can work particularly well for boy–girl pairs, who often drift apart around puberty. Another important factor is that girls tend to mature (in all senses of the word) much earlier than boys. There are still many single-sex schools, both within and outside the state system, and on the whole if there is one for girls in your area, there is often one of a similar standard and ethos for boys nearby too.

> Alexis goes to the girls' grammar school while Jasper goes to the boys' one, which is pretty much equivalent in terms of standards and is half a mile away from the girls' school. It is ideal for them (and me) because they come home on the same bus. The only bone of contention is that by the time the bus gets to Jasper's school, all the seats are taken by the girls.

For multiples of very different ability, and perhaps also for those of very similar appearance, separate schools with their different emphasis can help each child fulfil his potential and blossom without the constraint of his twin.

· *Selective Schools* ·

Some schools are selective, with admission depending on a child's performance in a test or series of tests and often on an interview as well. In the case of selective schools, especially independent schools, it is worth asking what the policy is regarding siblings. Most independent schools do not automatically give any preference to siblings. However, at the moment it is also fair to say that many private schools are experiencing a decline in the number of children applying. There may therefore be some leeway here if your children aren't strictly speaking of the same standard but you want them to attend the same selective school.

The situation is not uniform across the State sector either. A few local authorities won't separate twins into different schools, even when their scores at twelve plus are very different. Other local authorities do the opposite, separating twins when one has reached the required score to get into the selective school and the other has narrowly missed it.

If your twins perform differently and you want them both to go to the same selective school, you do have to consider first whether this would be in the best interests of each child as well as being more convenient. Naturally, academic results are important, but they are hardly ever the only factor in choosing schools. If you believe there are good reasons for your twins to be together (or apart) despite their exam results, say so. You can also ask TAMBA for support in this. Remember that the people you deal with at the education department or in the individual schools may not have had much experience of multiples – and they may have had no experience at all of multiples just like yours.

· *Choosing Secondary Schools* ·

Few areas are so isolated as to offer no alternatives and you will need to evaluate several factors in choosing schools.

1   The school itself

There are many different types of school – a huge topic which is outside the scope of this book – but how does one make a choice? How, for that matter, do you reach any decision regarding your children's future? The trouble is that you never can know all the facts in advance, but you can start by going to open evenings – with your children – and see what you think. Ask the staff how twins are dealt with. Think about the atmosphere of the school. Do you and your children like it? If you disagree, why is this?

You can also ask other parents in your area about local schools. However, beware of inaccurate gossip, which abounds about every school and is sometimes useless, especially if it is years out of date.

Scan league tables of exam results if you feel so inclined, although even enthusiasts of league tables agree that they do not give the whole picture. As an obvious example, schools with no sixth form will have no scores for A level. However, the main drawback of the tables is undoubtedly that they do not take into account the ability of the pupils admitted, so they do not (yet) reflect the 'value-added' factor.

2   The logistics

Under this heading fit all the obvious practical considerations, such as distance, travel time and perhaps finances. You might, for example, have considered private education, but have difficulty in affording two lots of school fees. In this case, investigate the assisted-places scheme and scholarships (though these last rarely cover more than a fraction of the fees these days).

3   The children

It is hard always to do the best thing for your children, especially when there are two or more of the same age. If your twins have been together throughout primary school, you may not have an entirely accurate picture of how each functions independently. For each child, you will need to think carefully about his:

- academic ability
- motivation
- interests
- independence from his twin
- social maturity
- need for privacy (often very great in multiples)
- any learning difficulties or special needs
- similarity in appearance to his twin.

Perhaps it is wrong to judge by physical appearance, but it is a fact that people do. It can also affect behaviour; playing tricks in which identical twins impersonate each other is an obvious example.

Your twins should have some say in the matter of their education. Of course, children should not have the privilege – or the burden – of making the final decision as to which school they go to, but their views and wishes do matter. Are they keen to be apart (or together)? What do they think of the particular schools under consideration? Where are their friends going to be?

One large school with six parallel classes was going to allocate one of two identical eleven-year-olds to a class where both had friends from primary school, while his twin would have been in a class where he knew nobody. A word in the head teacher's ear soon changed things. Without too much difficulty, each twin was placed in a class where he knew four or five of his peers.

· *Important Issues at Secondary School* ·

Little formal research has been carried out on multiples at secondary school, but a great deal of anecdotal evidence from twins, their parents and teachers suggests that certain issues crop up from time to time.

Identity

In school uniform, identical twins may resemble each other so closely that teachers have a great deal of trouble telling them apart. There may be a few centimetres difference in height, or one may have more freckles, but this is of no use when only one twin is present! If people have to ask who the child is before they are sure, so that every conversation starts with: 'Which one are you?' then individuality and sensitivity are obviously compromised and communications are the poorer for it.

By the time multiples get to secondary school, it is important that each should be able to function independently and have a strong sense of their own identity, which most do. However, the security and comfort of being a twin has a particular appeal, especially to a child who is shy, retiring or a little less able. This occasionally creates problems. In some pairs, one twin may continue to make the executive decisions while the other hangs back uncertainly.

At secondary school, some twins have been known to conceal their twinship, perhaps in an attempt to break free. Two non-identical boys who went to different schools did this very effectively for nearly two years, without either mentioning to anyone that he had a brother, let alone a twin.

Privacy

This is an issue throughout childhood and the teen years, but it has particular relevance to school. If your twins are at the same school, albeit in separate classes, you may find that one child tells you all about her twin: 'Natalie had to go see Mrs Worthington again,' 'Natalie fancies Roderick' and so on. Of course, not all twins tell tales on each other, but when they do, you can bet Natalie will get fed up with it.

Privacy over school life is essential – no child has a right to know his twin's results and still less to blurt them out as soon as he gets half-way through the front door. Whether the news is good or less good, each child should have his moment to share it with his parents in private. Whether multiples should see each other's reports varies from family to family. Obviously the children should only do so if they agree, a point which also applies to exam results.

> Alex had let Kim hear the marks on his end-of-year report, but Kim wasn't reciprocating because his own report, although very good, wasn't quite as glowing. Both boys ended up hopping mad.

Each child also needs a private place to work, and to do nothing if he chooses, away from the prying eyes of a sibling with Scotland Yard tendencies. Separate bedrooms are ideal, but not every family can provide that luxury. Some sort of partition across a bedroom can work, though it has occasionally been known for a dividing curtain to get pulled down in anger.

Behaviour

Boisterous children settle down eventually, but naughtiness can persist into secondary school and 'twin-power' may make it hard to handle. Sometimes one twin is wayward and the other meekly follows suit to avoid feeling left out. The end result is much the same and both end up in trouble.

Sometimes clowning around and other disruptive behaviour in class – or just inattention and lack of concentration –

emerge only when the twins come together for certain lessons after they have become used to being taught separately for a year or more. It may be an involuntary reaction to the chemistry of being together again, but occasionally it is a deliberate ploy to secure attention from teacher or classmates.

Homework

Even when they are in different classes or at different schools, twins may well be given similar homework, if only because of the content of the National Curriculum. It may be tempting to let them help each other, but this can be counter-productive. Each must learn to work independently.

There is scope for some compromise in certain areas, for instance sharing books for a project. Oddly enough, though, this is when some multiples argue the most fiercely!

> One of them got three library books on forestry and his brother only found one. Each guarded his jealously and we were treated to tantrums the like of which we hadn't seen for years.

However, they can work well together. Several mothers have told me that their twins help each other out. Twin-power can be a good thing when practising French conversation, or testing each other, but there is a danger here according to one mother (who is also a teacher):

> It's very tempting just to let them get on with it, but I know that, although they have each other, parents still need to be involved with schoolwork and show an interest.

On the other hand, when the homework load is distributed unequally between the children (perhaps because of different teaching styles) this can create problems. Officially there may be three homework subjects a night, but it may not always work out that evenly. The one with more homework on any one evening is likely to see this as grossly unfair and may fail to complete it, or else rush through it so he can join his twin slumped in front of the telly.

Different abilities

As at primary school, a disparity in ability can cause intense jealousy between twins, not to mention a lot of heartache for their parents. Most of us, consciously or not, still expect twins to be just the same in so many spheres.

The drawbacks of comparing multiples have already been covered in Chapters 8 and 11. This can continue to cause misery at secondary school and is sometimes accentuated by the physical and emotional turmoil of puberty, especially when each twin goes through puberty at a different time.

We are not all the same, but everyone has some talent. In the case of a less able child, this must be discovered so that his energy and enthusiasm can be channelled and his self-respect nurtured.

Different abilities can be a positive factor and make it easier to treat twins as individuals, at least where homework and careers advice are concerned, but there are times when it can hurt:

> Matthew got picked for the school football team and Andrew didn't, even though he thought he was the better player. He obviously wasn't, and he was gutted. But he got over it eventually and he now plays hockey.

Sports and music are obvious outlets for extra-curricular energies, but not the only ones. In one pair of non-identical boys, one brother was both more able and much more athletic. His twin did not appear to be good at anything until he discovered sleight of hand. Now his small build and newly found capacity for making jokes make him a popular amateur magician who specializes in entertaining at younger children's parties.

Exams

The strain of revising for and sitting exams is very stressful for any child. With twins, a double dose of 'exam crisis' can seriously affect the whole family. And then there are the results. One must of course congratulate anyone who has done well, even if this seems unfair because one twin gets most of the praise. It would be less fair to treat them equally if their efforts were unequal. After all, you don't want to heap praise on the one who has done a lot less work.

For those children who feel their results must be as good as their twin's, the pressure to achieve may be enormous. If they are of different aptitudes it may be impossible. GCSEs and A levels create particularly trying times. With some pairs, even minor differences in performance become magnified out of all proportion, leading to envy, sulking or guilt. They should have got over such feelings by the time they get to GCSEs, and most have, but not all.

One girl learned from the notice-board that she had excellent A-level results, but her heart sank because she was worried about her twin sister's marks. She felt guilty since she knew her sister couldn't have done as brilliantly.

For this reason, some twins try hard not to do too well. There may also be an element of inverted snobbery: a few teenagers, boys in particular, consider it 'uncool' to succeed academically.

Though they may seem interminable, exams do eventually end. As one parent says, 'Results arrive, for better or for worse. One lives through it, and life moves on.'

Teachers' attitudes

As a parent, one expects teachers to be experts in all aspects of education, but this is not always the case. Like all professionals – lawyers, doctors, and so on – teachers have their own interests and they are not all equally gifted in every subject or with every pupil.

Many teachers have had little or no training in the issues facing multiples at school. As at primary level, parents have to be prepared to co-operate closely and to point teachers in the right direction, preferably gently and tactfully (you catch more bears with honey). TAMBA provides useful study days and other resources for teachers.

· *Choices for the Future* ·

There is little published work in this area, and no hard and fast rules for parents. It would be easier if your twins went their separate ways during and after school and made different career choices. Then nobody would compare them again, or judge their performance relative to each other.

> It came as a shock to me when we were posted abroad to find that only one of our sixteen-year-old sons was planning on joining us. His brother wanted to go to boarding school back home and concentrate on his music. I don't think I was prepared for such a sudden and total separation, but if I'm honest I've always known they had different inclinations. And I'm proud that Mark felt able to make that decision.

However, many twins do choose the same subjects for their GCSEs and A levels. Some are genuinely interested in the same things. For example, one twin, now in middle age, lectures in Japanese at Oxford while his identical twin is professor of Chinese at Cambridge. Both also do work on Eastern religions. After all, many non-twin siblings share interests too and there is no shortage of children who follow in a parent's footsteps.

While helping each of your offspring to be individuals, it is important not to separate them forcibly. Different options for GCSE and A level may lead to a great deal of unhappiness if chosen for the wrong reasons. As for any youngster, it is essential for twins to make choices which are appropriate for them rather than because they suit someone else's agenda. There is, however, an element of chance and timing in selecting colleges and universities; sometimes it just depends on who got their form in first.

So if your children seem to want the same career, instead of trying to get them to change their minds, aim to find out why. Have they explored all their options? Are they indeed similar in their interests? Or are they afraid of leading adult lives which are too separate? If they have had good opportunities so far, this is unlikely to be the case. However, separate colleges or universities can be very traumatic if your twins have never been apart before.

Twins needn't necessarily drift away from each other because they attend different colleges or pursue different vocations. Even multiples at very distant universities may continually phone each other and spend more spare time and holidays together than they do with their parents. It could be a relief not to have all their dirty socks to wash at weekends, but some parents and siblings of twins can feel a bit left out and may take a while to get adjusted.

· *What Can Parents Do?* ·

Some parents of secondary-school children throw up their hands in horror, believing it is too late to change their children. In one or two ways perhaps that's true, but you can still usefully apply some of the ideas from the previous chapter. In fact you may not have to do much at all: many twins are well adjusted to functioning independently and have no problems, for example learning difficulties: they sail through secondary school without major hiccups. As some parents find, even identical twins tend to diverge more and more in the teen years and end up delightfully different. All you have to do is take the credit.

If you haven't already, try to:

- provide as much privacy as possible for each child
- provide as much space as possible (own desk, own room or whatever you can manage)
- encourage them not to compete for marks, friends, etc.
- treat them as individuals – no calling out for 'the Twinnies' when one of them is wanted at the door
- be sympathetic and supportive: let each of them tell you how she feels
- find something each is good at, but don't force them into separate choices just for the sake of it – multiples, and especially identicals, may genuinely have the same interests
- avoid getting upset if they play the odd trick of impersonating each other, as long as it is not in class
- go easy on unimportant issues: some things which make you see red now may not matter a bit in a year from now
- avoid making comparisons at all costs; especially try not to discipline one twin by complaining that his brother is always so much better behaved!
- agree with them when they complain that life's unfair – it is, and it's a tough lesson to learn.

· *Parents' Evenings* ·

These can be something of an endurance test for parents of multiples; even those who only have singletons find it hard to whizz round trying to see all the teachers in one evening and remember what was said. Here are some suggestions from parents of twins about making it work:

- Take a notebook and pencil. You may just remember what six different teachers said about one child (and the points you want to raise), but with twins or more you will definitely need something to jog your memory.

- If you have a partner, perhaps he could see one child's teachers while you deal with those of the other twin.

- Go on two separate evenings if you can, or arrange to see some teachers at another time, perhaps just before or after classes one schoolday.

- If you cannot see all the staff, concentrate on meeting the teachers who seem most vital for each child. You could explain your predicament to the school in advance and ask their advice as to whom you really must see on Parents' Evening.

- Even if your children have the same teachers, always stick to discussing one child at a time, as at primary school. (Much of the other advice given in Chapter 11 is still useful at secondary level.)

Chapter Thirteen

ADOLESCENCE AND THE TEEN YEARS

Adolesco is Latin for 'I grow up.' Adolescence, the process of becoming an adult, can put years on the parents too. When my own twins reached their first birthday, I could finally foresee an end to the round-the-clock demands of babycare and I recall confidently telling a friend that with twins the first year was the worst. Being the father of twins himself, he disagreed. 'With twins,' he replied, 'the first twenty years are the worst.'

It was said in jest, but contains a grain of truth. For many parents of twins adolescence is a time when their children grow further apart and rebel against the twinship. This can be something of a sea change for parents, who often cease to be seen as parents of twins at this stage. Some will miss this and look back wistfully to the time when their twins were just babies.

Meanwhile, the adolescent twin is faced not just with breaking away from parental control but also with separating from his co-twin. All the evidence suggests that the earlier in life this process starts, and the more used each child has become to being treated as an individual in his own right, the easier adolescence is. But, however exemplary your raising of your twins has been so far, you cannot rely on having an easy ride in the teen years. In fact, you can't count on anything much during these sometimes painful years.

Perhaps the essence of puberty is that feelings are deeply ambiguous. While on the one hand twins may rebel against the twinship, on the other hand they still value its special bond.

· *What Adolescence is Like* ·

The teen years tend to be difficult even for singletons. There may be no such thing as growing pains, but, as the eminent paediatrician John Apley put it, 'Physical growth does not hurt, though emotional growth can hurt like hell!' If you can't remember your own teenage years in all their awfulness, bear in mind that they are a time of enormous hormonal and emotional upheaval and coincide with increasing educational and social pressures.

- Teenagers are very critical of themselves. One single spot can be a disaster of national significance. They also tend to be highly critical of others and especially of the adult world.

- They need approval, but as a parent you should beware of how you give it. The average teenager doesn't want his mother to think he looks 'very smart, dear' – he'd much rather look like his peers, in other words like some unspeakable creature from the Blue Lagoon.

- Teenagers may be despondent about the future. True depression does occur in this age group, but many more youngsters are simply worried about the rest of their lives (and perhaps with good reason, given current employment prospects).

- Adolescents are very changeable from one minute to the next. Not all are, of course, but the see-saws in ideas and emotions can seem violent.

- Teenagers tend to be very territorial and you may hear each of your twins talking much more about '*My* room', '*My* CDs' or whatever.

- Perhaps it is the raging hormones that make teenagers so intense, reacting to even minor irritants. Whatever the reason, the most trivial things can end up getting on their nerves – and yours too, of course.

- Meanwhile, they are bombarded from all sides by images and messages which suggest they ought to be good-looking, super-cool, slim and so on.

- Adolescence comes at a time when many parents find it especially hard to cope. If your twins were born when you were 35, which is far from unusual, during most of their teen years you will be in your fifties, and possibly coping with the difficulties of the menopause, redundancy or forthcoming retirement.

- Divorce rates are continuing to rise, so you may be caring for teenaged twins on your own, with all the practical and emotional burdens that single parenthood entails.

· *Some Practical Problems of* · *Teenaged Twins*

Puberty

Twins (and triplets) often mature at different times. It is normal for girls to go through puberty two years ahead of boys. This is often when the girl of a mixed-sex pair will be both more mature in looks and attitude, as well as taller than her twin because she has already had her adolescent growth spurt and he has not. Between the ages of eleven and thirteen, she may be both taller and look more grown-up than her twin brother.

Same-sex pairs, and even identical twins, can also go through puberty at different times, however, as paediatrician Dr John Buckler confirms. There may be an interval of six months or a year before they both reach the same physical stage. This has many implications:

- If twins appear to be of different ages, the outward signs of twinship are in effect lost.

- The effect of looking more mature is that people expect you to behave in a more adult way.

- Those who mature later (especially boys) seem to suffer more crises of confidence.

- Puberty makes one highly sensitive about one's body. Pubertal twins desperately need privacy, all the more so if they're at different developmental stages.

- An adolescent twin can become acutely aware of being less attractive (or less well-endowed) than his or her same-sex twin.

Identity

Self-esteem depends crucially on identity – doesn't every adolescent try to 'find himself'? Even if they have been happy looking alike, in adolescence twins often consider it important to appear different. If they have always shared some clothes before, now is the time when it becomes anathema. (This is one good reason why twins should have their own clothes from early childhood.)

They may not always succeed. One father comments: 'My daughters think they're dressing differently, but they're both in black denim jeans all the time and it may as well be a uniform.'

In an attempt to look dissimilar, two identical girls of seventeen each went to the hairdresser's separately and asked for their lovely long hair to be cut, simply requesting a style that suited them. They ended up with exactly the same bob.

Independence

In a same-sex pair, the dominant twin may continue to make all the decisions and take the lead, to the detriment of his twin's development. The dominant one is often (though not necessarily) the one who is more advanced physically.

Dominance may change in adolescence. Sometimes one wants to break free, while the other doesn't – a situation which can be as painful as the break-up of any relationship. It is often the less dominant twin who wants freedom from his sibling in the teen years. Meanwhile, the hitherto dominant partner may begin to feel insecure without the constant presence and quiet support of his twin.

In girl–boy pairs, the boy may become protective of his twin sister, acting as her chaperone and perhaps even her moral custodian, although she may resent it. Or she may find her brother's presence distinctly advantageous: you may allow her to stay out later or go to places you would have tried to forbid her from going had she been on her own. As one girl recalls: 'My brother was often at the same parties and our parents thought that was great. But then, they didn't know that he was legless most of the time.'

Whether they're the same sex or not, allowing twins to go out together can be convenient – surely there is safety in numbers? This is not always best for their individual development and may inhibit one or both. One of a set of identical girls was always the leader, going around with a wild, rebellious crowd who frequently got into trouble. Not wishing to be left behind, her far more introverted sister just tagged along, unhappy to be with them, yet unhappy on her own.

Friendships

Several people, including family therapist Audrey Sandbank, have pointed out that twins often start dating later than singletons: no bad thing, you may think, since children seem to grow up so soon these days. This is probably a reflection of the fact that twins have each other for company and hence less immediate need of others. But the time will come.

It can be awkward making friends, of either sex. Many parents of teenaged twins comment that, although their children have lots of friends, they do not have one or two very close ones. Perhaps outsiders are reluctant to intrude on the special relationship twins often have. When one of them does have a best friend, intense jealousy can result, with the other twin feeling left out or perhaps trying to muscle in and share the best friend.

· Single-Parent Issues ·

It is demanding enough for two parents to deal with the ups and downs of one teenager, so how does one adult alone cope with two or more adolescents?

Those who head single-parent families may find it very tough bringing up children without a resident role model of the opposite gender. There can be many other practical and financial problems when you are on your own: single parents may be lonely, isolated socially and in reduced circumstances.

It is hard for a lone parent to have the conviction to support his or her own point of view without the reinforcement and feedback of a partner. In the case of twins, it can be particularly difficult to be consistent and firm when faced with an onslaught of demands from more than one awkward adolescent. No wonder there are times when it is much easier just to give in and say 'yes' rather than 'no' to two or more stroppy teenagers.

On the other hand, the juggling act that single parents have to become adept at has its rewards. Consistency in handling your children is less of a problem – after all, there is no one to undermine you or persuade you to overturn your decisions!

Children of lone parents, far from running wild, are often quite mature in their emotions, very supportive of their parent and able to show a great deal of understanding. Single-parent households are frequently noted for the closeness of the parent–child relationship and families of twins are no exception. As a single parent comes through this difficult time, he or she may often feel a great deal of pride in the twins and of course in having reared them alone. But it can be painful to let the youngsters go.

TAMBA's One-Parent Families Group offers information and support from other members.

· *What Can Parents Do to Help* · *Adolescents?*

All youngsters are different and to some extent adolescence is uncharted territory, but there are some ways of making things easier:

- Avoid labelling your twins (not that you would even dream of it any more, would you?)

- Give each twin as much privacy as you can provide. This includes emotional privacy, the security of knowing he can be listened to without his twin being there or hearing all about it later. Watch out for teenagers who eavesdrop.

- Don't take advantage of the twin relationship. For many years, your children may have understood each other intuitively (one of mine often said, 'Ask me – I know Oliver better than anyone else does'), but in adolescence and beyond it is important to resist asking one effectively to tell on the other.

- Try not to assume that they will look out for each other's physical or emotional welfare. It is not necessarily a youngster's fault that his twin is upset.

- Allow your twins to work out their own relationship. There are many advantages to having a twin and you may be able to help your teenagers by emphasizing the positive side of twinship. However, try not to fall into the trap of envying them. You are unlikely to win anyone over by saying, 'If only I'd had a twin sister at your age I'd have *loved* it, not complained about it constantly.'

- Don't assume that your twins still have the same likes and dislikes. Even if they're identical, adolescence is a time when their tastes can diverge dramatically. Don't automatically choose identical presents for them at Christmas.

- Many twins will want separate birthday parties at this age, on different days, with different guests. On the other hand, many do not mind sharing a birthday, contrary to what many parents may imagine. It is better to ask them than to make assumptions.

- Teenagers' self-esteem can be boosted if they are given more responsibility, such as a part-time job or a paper round. Twins may be ready to look after younger siblings – and to baby-sit for other families – at a slightly earlier age than singletons.

- Don't be critical or unnecessarily judgemental. Youngsters need rules, but it is best to give them as much leeway as you can, saving your anger for some really outrageous misbehaviour.

- If your children are still angelic, don't be fooled into thinking that they'll always be the heavenly twins. Their adolescent rebellion may just come a little later than it does for singletons.

- Finally, parents of teenaged twins strongly advise others to keep a sense of humour. Seeing the funny side can certainly help get everyone through adolescent traumas. Once they have grown up, you will no doubt feel a deep sense of achievement, though you may feel sad too. If you've always been at home, try to develop some new interests. It might also make you seem interesting to your children – you never know your luck.

Chapter Fourteen

SPECIAL SITUATIONS, SPECIAL NEEDS

Having twins, like being a twin, is generally a joyful business despite its challenges. Many a mother has jollied herself along through trying times with her multiples with the thought that she can put up with almost anything as long as the children are healthy.

Sadly, there are circumstances in which one or other twin is handicapped to some extent, or does not survive. It is to their families that this chapter is addressed. Not every special need can be covered here, but I hope there will be something to help most parents facing such a situation.

· *Special Needs* ·

Although the vast majority of multiple-birth children are completely healthy, the overall rate of disability is greater in twins and higher multiples than in singletons. The main reasons are:

- prematurity
- poor growth in the womb ('small for dates' infants)
- sometimes, complications of pregnancy (e.g. twin-to-twin transfusion syndrome and pre-eclampsia)
- advances in neonatal care which increase the survival of vulnerable babies who, once upon a time, might not have lived.

A few experts also suggest that the twinning process itself could be a factor implicated in some disabilities in identical (MZ) twins. This is possible, though the theory is still speculative at this point.

Different kinds of disabilities

As with all other children, the range of disability which can affect twins is very wide, from trivial to severe and from rare to fairly frequent. While some conditions are so unusual that they affect only a small number of families in the entire country, there are other more common disabilities, including:

- cerebral palsy (the risk is believed to be three times higher in twins and perhaps ten times higher in triplets)
- various congenital heart defects, such as ventricular or atrial septal defects ('hole in the heart') and transposition of the great vessels
- delayed mental development or learning difficulties.

When one twin, even of an identical pair, has a disability caused by an inborn abnormality, very often his twin does not. Discordance is the medical term for this situation. Its opposite, concordance, means that both twins have the same condition. However, concordant twins aren't necessarily affected to exactly the same degree: one twin can be healthier than the other.

Surprisingly, discordance is usual in otherwise identical twins, especially in congenital heart disease. Even some hereditary conditions like muscular dystrophy do not always affect both youngsters, so that patently identical twins are not strictly identical. One theory which could explain some abnormalities is that the splitting of the fertilized egg to form identical twins has an effect on midline organs (like the heart, gullet, etc.). Perhaps this is because one twin ends up with fewer cells from the splitting.

Effects on the family

Whatever the nature or the underlying cause, disability in a twin can affect the whole family. The presence of a healthy twin often means that a problem is picked up sooner than it might otherwise have been. For instance, a delay in one baby in starting to talk or crawl is particularly obvious when the other one is developing in leaps and bounds.

Clearly, the effects go far deeper. When only one twin is handicapped, the presence of a healthier sibling of exactly the same age can be a poignant and sometimes painful reminder of what might have been – or, as some parents say, of what should have been.

The parents

Losing, as it were, the health of a child is a form of bereavement. There may also be grief over the apparent loss of the twinship. Many parents comment on how painful it is for them to come across pairs of able-bodied twins and some go to great lengths to avoid it if they can.

Some mothers feel their loss of status as a parent of twins very acutely. While a few continue to go to great lengths to preserve outward appearances of twin-ness (with identical clothes, for instance), others prefer not to remind themselves or outsiders of the twinship. The comparisons which seem to be an almost inevitable aspect of twinship can be too hard to bear.

The parents of a disabled child may feel intensely guilty or angry. These emotions are perhaps irrational and even unproductive, but understandable none the less. The anger directed at medical professionals can be all the greater when multiples resulted from fertility treatment.

Sometimes parents may find it hard to believe that the remaining healthy twin or triplets are all right. Especially in the early days, the well children are sometimes taken repeatedly to the doctor's, just to make sure. However, this eventually stops – the parents either come to believe that the child is healthy or are simply kept too busy attending to the sick one's needs.

The burden of caring for a disabled youngster is obviously far greater when he is one of multiples, because there is already so much to do. When both twin babies are handicapped, a mother (and it usually is the mother) may find it impossible to cope. Inevitably, little time is left for the parents to spend with each other. Shortage of time and energy, and often money too, leads to severe restrictions on what a family can do. The logistic problems can result in social isolation. This is hard for any parent, but especially, perhaps, for a mother who has until now had her own career.

Much of the help given to a family with special needs is aimed at the affected children and their mother. Fathers tend to become marginalized, although they have needs as well. Even if he is hesitant to express himself, a father too can feel angry, guilty, cheated or overwhelmed. He may have even more anxieties than his partner: as one mother explained, her husband rarely got a chance to go to the special school, or see the doctors, to find out just how well their handicapped son was doing. A father needs to be involved from the early days and to receive support in a form he finds acceptable.

Some parents of disabled twins do, it seems, physically abuse their children, especially if only one twin is handicapped. This can only make a difficult situation worse. Cruelty to children is hard to understand and easy to condemn, but those of us with healthy offspring cannot appreciate what the pressures are like.

The healthy twin

Parents of one disabled twin often go to great lengths to be fair to both children. This is especially difficult since time is so short and, whatever they do, it may simply not seem enough. It is inevitable that the healthier of the two will get less attention, but the child may not see it that way. Why should his brother's first syllable or faltering step be so ecstatically acclaimed, while he has been doing far more than this for absolutely ages without a word of praise?

The healthier twin may indulge in showing off or other forms of attention-seeking, or he may regress until (not surprisingly) his behaviour comes to resemble that of his disabled twin.

Later on, the healthy twin sometimes feels guilty, not simply for his own awkward behaviour but perhaps for his twin's condition, as if he were in some way responsible for it. He may just feel guilty about being the healthy survivor, or he may be under pressure to help care for his twin (though he should never have to).

Some healthy siblings are remarkably well-adjusted and take it all in their stride, however:

> I've done my best to be fair, but I know I haven't always succeeded. Inevitably I spend far more time and effort on my sick twin, who has needed heart surgery several times. As far as David (the healthy one) is concerned, he's accepted it and he's been brilliant. But then he's never known any different.

If one twin is disabled, he is automatically different. It may be an advantage in these circumstances if neither he nor his co-twin thinks of himself as a twin:

> We never discouraged Robert from thinking of himself as a twin, but we never harped on about it either. He just never particularly regarded himself as in any way twinned with his brother, apart from having to share a birthday. They've been different from the word go in all sorts of ways, physically and because of Gavin's gullet problem and his learning difficulties.

In this case, Robert is quite supportive of his less able brother, but some twins are acutely embarrassed by their twin's medical condition. They may indeed prefer to conceal the twinship from their friends.

A few healthy twins learn to grow up fast. They should never have to be responsible for the special-needs twin. However, they sometimes take on tasks more suitable for an older child and can become very protective of the less able twin. Again, the difference between the fit child and the sick one is an obvious factor here. Perhaps it is also significant that the healthier one is often looked after by various friends or relatives, while the handicapped one gets Mum. Sometimes being, in effect, farmed out results in clinginess, but in other cases the child swiftly learns about separation.

For practical reasons, outings are often restricted. Even with appropriate access, a visit to a museum may be unsuitable for the disabled child, something the healthy twin is likely to resent. For many years the only outings may be tedious protracted outpatient visits, tagging along with his handicapped sibling.

A healthy twin may be desperate to go to Disney World like his school friends, but this may be out of the question for the time being at least. Holidays are often restricted to short breaks nearer home and even then can be anything but restful. One family with special-needs triplets always made sure they chose a campsite near a hospital with an accident and emergency department.

The work of special schools, MBF and TAMBA shows that the special needs of the healthy twin are not always recognized, let alone consistently met. To focus on the issues facing the healthy twin, paediatricians Christine Burton and Elizabeth Bryan of the MBF carried out a survey of parents of only one disabled twin.

They found that most parents had little trouble explaining

the disability to the healthy sibling, but that there were enormous difficulties in dealing with it. The overwhelming majority of parents believed that the disability had affected the well child and that he often received less attention, and at times fewer presents too.

The healthy twin sometimes had problems, either behavioural difficulties (feeding, sleeping, tantrums, etc.) or physical ailments like asthma and eczema. Because of the small size of the survey, it is impossible to know whether these are significantly more common in twins with a disabled co-twin, but they might be.

On occasion, friends and professionals who came to the house virtually ignored the healthy one. One or two parents commented that professionals weren't understanding about the significance of the twinship. One paediatrician had apparently told a mother of one twin with cerebral palsy that being a twin 'shouldn't make any difference'.

The findings of this survey suggest that some professionals could do better and also point the way for further useful work into the long-term effects on a family of having a multiple with special needs.

· *Getting Help* ·

Not all is gloom and doom for special-needs families, as the following shows:

> My triplets – all girls – were born at 27 weeks and were seriously ill in special care for over three months each. Our older daughter Katie was three years old at the time, and we included her in everything. She took it on board – her dolls often had cardiac arrests, and she'd put them on ventilators made of Duplo bricks. People were horrified, but it was her way of coping. Now it is nine years on. The triplets all have special needs but all four girls are well adjusted and play

nicely together. Even in the bleakest days, when I was told one or more would die, I was hopeful and kept hanging on. Now I count myself lucky.

There can even be benefits when one twin has special needs. The disabled twin is stimulated and encouraged by his constant companion and has a role model to emulate, while the healthier twin often gains in insight, empathy and understanding. All the same, nobody would actually wish for all the difficulties that disability in the family can bring.

Families with one or more multiples with special needs require information about the disability itself, financial and practical assistance and long-term emotional and social support. Help is at hand from various groups and agencies.

Doctors and other professionals play an obvious role in arranging such things as specialist referrals, physiotherapy, special diets and adaptations to the home (for instance through occupational therapists). While many doctors also form the backbone of support for a family, some are not very good at explaining the disability itself – its nature, causes, and long-term outlook.

> The paediatrician just announced, 'I think one of your twins has got Down's syndrome.' Then he left the room. What did he mean 'think'? I needed to *know*. I also needed to know what would become of James and what kind of life he'd have. The staff nurse wasn't encouraging. She told me to expect him to be no more than a vegetable. Fortunately, that's not the case at all. Both he and his twin start at a normal school this year.

The wide variety of patient groups – from Arthritis Care to the Williams Syndrome Foundation – do an excellent job of providing information in an accessible form. In many cases they also help support the family with a sympathetic ear, a network of local groups and information on the various benefits and allowances they may qualify for.

Support groups play an additional role in raising public and professional awareness and stimulating (and often funding) medical research.

As soon as they can, parents should contact the appropriate support group, but this is not always possible. In some instances, no firm diagnosis is given, or the family is told that the child's diagnosis is so rare that there are only a few sufferers in the country and they are unlikely ever to meet another child with the same disorder. For these, the national charity Contact-a-Family (see page 344) is an invaluable resource, helping families whose children have a rare or undiagnosed condition.

Within TAMBA, the Special Needs Group exists specifically to support families with one or more multiples who have disabilities. This committed group, run by parents, produces a regular newsletter with advice and views, and creates a contact network for those who want to get in touch with others in a similar situation. TAMBA also provides immediate telephone advice via TAMBA Twinline (see page 343).

The MBF welcomes special-needs families and their paediatricians can often see them at sessions of their twins clinics.

There is also a huge annual special-needs party (with entertainment), which families from all over the country enjoy. One child was heard to say that he wants to attend every year until he's 'really old'. The party is also much appreciated by the healthy twin and parents. At first, many parents are not aware how much help and equipment are available, and they often learn a great deal from each other. You can find out more from MBF or TAMBA Special Needs Group.

Many families with handicapped twins benefit from the support of friends, relatives and voluntary workers. One mother tells of her good fortune in meeting another family who had twins one year older with the same condition:

I knew that whatever difficulties I faced, there was someone else I could talk to who not only knew what it was like, but had lived through exactly that stage already – and survived.

· *Special Educational Needs* ·

A fairly common situation is where one or other school-aged twin has special educational needs. Along with the new Education Act 1993 which applies to England and Wales, there has been since September 1994 a Code of Practice which gives guidance to schools, education authorities and others on how best to identify, assess and provide for pupils with special educational needs.

The needs a child has could be mild or severe, temporary or permanent, but must be addressed so that the child can benefit as much as possible from education generally and the National Curriculum in particular. The entire process emphasizes partnership between parents and the agencies and professionals involved; an important principle embodied in the code of practice is that the parents' wishes should be taken into account. It does not necessarily follow that their wishes will be granted, however. Since September 1994, parents have been able to appeal to an independent body, the Special Educational Needs tribunal, but the process can take a long time and is sometimes expensive.

For a child with special educational needs, there are several stages of assessment, starting with the point at which concern is raised. The concern might be about anything from poor counting to disruptive behaviour – and, incidentally, gifted youngsters are also considered to have special educational needs.

In England and Wales, every State school (and a number of independent schools) has access to an educational psychologist and in the process of assessing your child's needs you may be asked to give consent for your child to see one. Unfortunately, most educational psychologists have no special training in dealing with multiples. As a minimum, twins and higher multiples should be assessed on different days and the reports about them written on different days too.

It is not often possible for the educational psychologist to see your twin or twins regularly and you may need to involve other resources, for instance family therapy. You can get guidance on educational issues from TAMBA.

You may have heard of 'statementing'. This refers to a statement of special educational needs, a term which, educational psychologists sometimes remind us, shouldn't be used as a verb at all. Briefly, a statement of special educational needs describes the problem in question (along with any non-educational needs), identifies the objectives and outlines the provision to be made to meet them. As a parent, you have the chance to read the statement and comment on it.

A statement of special educational needs carries no stigma or long-term implication. It doesn't label a child so much as define his needs in an attempt to meet them. Even so, some parents worry about a statement, or about the fact that one of their twins may have been 'statemented' and not the other. If you are concerned about your child being demeaned, just ask yourself, what would be the implications of *not* getting help for his special educational needs?

· *When a Twin Dies* ·

The death of both twins is self-evidently a tragedy and it is easy to recognize it as one. We normally expect to live longer than our children, so, like all deaths in childhood, it is 'wrong' because it is the wrong way round.

> Both my twins died within fifteen hours of birth. For a long long time I felt something inside had died too. It was me.

The loss has to be lived through, worked though and ulti-mately, perhaps many years later, accepted – although, as the columnist Virginia Ironside has put it, you do not really work through bereavement. It works through you.

Tragic though the death of both twins is, it involves none of the conflicting emotions that parents endure when they lose one of their multiples and others survive.

The rest of this section focuses on the loss of one twin (or triplet), not because the death of both (or all) babies is any less important but because the difficulties for the family are different.

The death of one twin differs in several ways. First, the survivor acts as a constant reminder of the loss – and how can the family celebrate his life while coping with his twin's death? Second, he needs to be looked after by his parents, no matter how disabled they are by grief. Third, many well-meaning people fail to understand the extent of the parents' bereavement in these circumstances and often think that a mother who has lost a twin should be content to have one remaining child.

The growing work done in this field at MBF and else-where shows that the loss of one twin, far from being easier on the parents, as many people might expect, is made much harder to bear because of the need to carry on with daily life and especially with caring for the co-twin. This postpones the essential process of mourning, as when a pregnancy swiftly follows a still birth or infant death, only obviously more so.

Unfortunately, even those medical professionals who should be of most help to parents who lose one twin have been known to misunderstand, and make hurtful comments which betray an attitude of 'least said, soonest mended'. Not surprisingly, parents of a dead twin tend to talk less about their grief to professionals than do those who lose a singleton.

Yet these parents' needs may be greater. Research suggests that mothers who lose one newborn twin are at higher risk from mental ill-health a year later than those who lose their only child. Another recent study shows that a parent who loses a twin at birth is more likely to feel hostile, confused and angry than one who loses a singleton.

Part of the grief, according to bereaved parents, is due to the loss of the pride and specialness that goes with twins or higher multiples in the family. A mother, one of whose twins has died, continues to think of herself as a mother of twins, as Elizabeth Bryan has pointed out, and this may need to be acknowledged. Similarly, a mother of triplets one of whom has died is still a mother of triplets – she is not somehow 'demoted' to the rank of mother of twins.

Unresolved parental grief is hard on the surviving children, especially the co-twin, who also goes through complex emotional reactions (discussed later in this chapter). A grieving mother may find the demands of childcare overwhelming and be unable to give her best to the surviving twin, but grieve she and her partner must, going through the various stages in the ways which are most appropriate for them. If you are in this situation, the best advice would be not to underestimate the magnitude of your loss or try to rush the process.

James Hollis, a Jungian psychotherapist, writes in his book *The Middle Passage* that grief in general is the occasion for acknowledging the value of what has been experienced. Because it has been experienced, it cannot be wholly lost. It is there, says Hollis, retained in the bones and the memory, to serve and guide the life to come.

Experience of the dead twin seems to be an essential part of coming to terms with the loss. When a twin is stillborn or dies as a very young baby, the loss is no less real, but there will have been little opportunity to experience him in life. What then can one keep in the bones and the memory to respect both the child and the twinship?

Death before birth

Although there will have been little chance to create evidence of their baby before he died, there are still ways in which parents can mark his existence.

- You could have a photo reproduced from an ultrasound scan, preferably an early one when both babies were alive, but if not any scan that shows both together.

- Although staff might not think of it, you may want to see, and perhaps hold, the dead twin at delivery. If you and your partner want time alone with the baby, say so.

- Photographs or paintings often become treasured mementoes. Many firms can marry two or more separate photos so that a family group is created. When a twin dies long before delivery you may not consider photos to be suitable for showing to others, but sometimes an artist can produce an attractive composite sketch or painting from separate photographs of babies (or even fetuses).

- Naming the dead baby makes it easier for the family to talk about her. Perhaps you could avoid a name which too obviously matches the survivor's (e.g. Daisy and Rose).

- You may be able to arrange a funeral service.

- Even after the body has been disposed of, some priests are prepared to baptize stillborn babies (occasionally even babies who technically miscarried). This can be a great solace to parents. Strictly speaking, this is a baptism 'by intent', and the normal certificate of baptism is issued with those two words added.

- Some kind of memorial service can be held. It does not need to take place straight away – it can be many years hence.

- You could mark the existence of the twin in some other tangible way, for instance in the hospital's memorial book, or by planting a tree or inscribing a plaque.

- You and your partner shouldn't avoid discussing your baby together as a couple and with friends and relatives. In due course you will also need to talk to your surviving twin.

Most of these suggestions apply no matter when in pregnancy the twin's death occurred, although there is a particular complication with the death of one baby early in pregnancy. When a twin dies before 24 weeks (or is selectively terminated) while the other continues to term, legally this is considered a miscarriage. However, many parents find it comforting to have both babies registered as twins and this is often possible if you ask.

Death of a young baby or child

This often takes place in hospital, especially in the special care baby unit, where staff may be experienced in dealing with bereaved parents, though perhaps less adept at handling the death of one twin.

When a twin or higher multiple is dying, parents should be encouraged to spend as much time with this baby as possible. There will be plenty of time later with the surviving infant(s). Few staff appreciate this at the time and may suggest that a mother concentrate on the healthier of the two. Yet later parents often wish that they had held and looked after the sicker baby more, instead of letting a kindly nurse relieve them of his care.

There are many ways in which a parent can mark and commemorate the existence of the baby:

- Photographs help, preferably of both or all the babies together. Even after one has died, photos can be taken of them together if you want. There are few medical reasons why this should not be done. TAMBA's midwifery advisor Jane Spillman points out that, whereas this sometimes shocks nursing staff, parents don't usually find it macabre.

- Other useful mementoes are hospital wrist or ankle tags, cot cards, locks of hair and even footprints or fingerprints. You may not want to look at these right away, and may not even appreciate their value now, but as time passes items like these can become treasured possessions.

- Some hospitals have a memorial book in which to inscribe details of the baby.

- As always, naming the baby facilitates talking about him now and in the years to come, not least with the surviving twin when the time comes.

- If you have a same-sex pair, zygosity determination can enable you to know for sure whether they are identical (monozygotic). This can sometimes be arranged if you ask early on.

- Keeping in touch with hospital staff may be your only contact with people who knew your baby in life. Spillman notes that one parent returned to the hospital on his twins' birthday for five years after one of them had died.

Help for bereaved families

Many mothers who lose a baby or child are advised to get over it by trying again for another baby as soon as possible. However, pregnancy and birth, being the antitheses of death, inhibit proper mourning. Although the next baby is usually much cherished – and much worried about – rushing into another pregnancy tends to be a poor idea, even when the entire set of twins or triplets was lost.

Fortunately, help is available to families who lose one or all of their multiple-birth children. The TAMBA Bereavement Support Group (BSG) was set up by and for such families, including those who have suffered a cot death and those who go through complete loss of an assisted pregnancy. The BSG newsletter is a forum for views and many bereaved parents have found that writing for it has crystallized their feelings and helped them come to terms with events. In the evenings TAMBA Twinline takes calls from parents with a variety of queries, including those in the acute distress of bereavement.

MBF can offer telephone support to bereaved parents and also runs bereavement clinics. On clinic days, TAMBA BSG holds an informal lunch for anyone who wants to attend. Some parents only seek help years after losing a twin, but it seems that it is never too late to acknowledge such a loss.

As in most childcare issues, men tend to be sidelined or at least under-represented. Although help is offered to fathers too, mothers find it easier to avail themselves of it. Sometimes a father's reaction is at odds with his partner's over their loss, but either way it is hard for him to express how he feels. Even in these supposedly caring times, there are few acceptable ways for men to open up. Back at work, colleagues may not think of raising the topic with a bereaved father or asking how things are. Nor may he want to burden friends and family. After all, real men don't cry. Or do they?

· *The Surviving Twin* ·

Children feel emotions acutely and the long-term effects of death on a surviving child, especially the co-twin, can be devastating. The link between twins is often the strongest of all human bonds and it would be surprising if this were not the case.

Even those who lose a twin in very early childhood can be deeply affected. Strange as it may seem, a few people whose co-twin was stillborn have remarked that they'd always felt incomplete – long before they ever knew they were a twin. They tend to be relieved when they find out that they once had a twin, if only for a few months of life in the womb.

Experts agree that it is a mistake to try to shield a young-ster from a death in the family. Although a child's notion of dying may be unsophisticated, he must be told at some point that he both had and lost a twin, preferably before he hears it from someone else. Parents are often surprised at how well children accept this. The surviving child may be extraordinarily proud of the twinship; some like to share the news immediately with their best friend.

If a child is old enough at the time of death, the funeral or memorial service can provide an important way to say good-bye. Even very young children can get involved by playing their own special role – choosing a song to sing or putting a posy of flowers on the coffin. They should be allowed and encouraged to do so if they want, though they shouldn't be forced to.

Whatever the age at which his twin dies, the survivor may feel guilty. Sometimes it is because he feels he didn't look out for his twin, but it may just be non-specific guilt at having survived. As one girl says of her twin brother's still birth, she was not expected to live either – which is why, her parents told her, they deliberately gave her an ugly name.

Parents need to be careful not to say anything that could lay any blame on the survivor. It can take a great deal of thought to avoid mentioning overcrowding in the womb, lack of nourishment or, say, the suggestion that if Mum hadn't been distracted by Ben, Amy might not have run into the path of an oncoming car.

Any of these may well have happened, possibly colouring the parents' attitude and emotions. The survivor may feel worthless as well as guilty. This is particularly likely to happen when the survivor of a boy–girl pair is, as far as one or other parent is concerned, the 'wrong' sex.

As only half of the twin pair, a survivor may feel that his value is diminished. Sometimes parents idolize the dead twin, and unconsciously vilify the one who is still alive:

> Somehow I was made to feel second-rate, even before my brother died (at the age of five). He was always the sickly one, but never complained. I was healthy, lively, and too much trouble – at least from our mother's point of view. I realize now that things were tough for her. I was made to feel even worse after he died because she kept going on and on about how perfect he was, 'not like her'.

Of course, the survivor's misdemeanours can be only too obvious. The surviving child may be hard to handle when he's going through his own emotional maelstrom. In coping with his own grief and confusion he may do things his parents find distressing, such as talking to his dead twin, taking his place at the dining-table or eating only half the food put in front of him.

Occasionally the surviving twin himself seems to court death, especially if the process has been glorified in any way. One six-year-old boy persisted in standing in the road outside the house; perhaps it is significant that this happened around Easter. His twin had not died in an accident, but, as he explained, he wanted to die so Baby Jesus could take him to his brother.

Whatever caused the death, the mother sometimes demands frequent medical check-ups for the surviving child for fear of losing him too. In the case of an illness like leukaemia, it may seem incredible to parents that the remaining child has escaped his twin's fate – they wonder for how long. Sometimes such concerns are rational, but sometimes they are not.

The surviving child may need the expert help of a child psychiatrist, and referral to a traumatic stress clinic that specializes in youngsters can be appropriate. The parents also need help with their emotions. Left unresolved, their own grief will make things much harder on the child.

Death is rarely all over and done with, and it does not annul a twinship. Children usually benefit if the memory of their dead twin is kept alive and in later years are often grateful to their parents for this. Parents shouldn't discourage their children from talking about their dead twin. Some youngsters like to visit the grave at special times to place flowers there or just to think, but it takes tact to do this on appropriate anniversaries without spoiling the survivor's birthday celebrations.

At whatever age death occurred, and despite the parents' best efforts, some survivors still feel like only half of a whole. Perhaps this is a unique feature of twinship.

· *Lone Twins as Adults* ·

I believe that if you started life together, then you were meant to be together.

Research shows that bereaved children in general tend to have a higher risk of later psychiatric illness, especially depression. In the 1980s, psychotherapist Joan Woodward carried out a study specifically on surviving twins. She interviewed 219 adults, some of whom had lost a twin in childhood, while others had been bereaved more recently. Woodward herself had lost her identical sister Pamela at the age of three. Over 80 per cent of the twins in her study rated their response to their twin's death as having had a severe or marked effect on their lives. The death of identical or same-sex twins tended to have more severe consequences. Perhaps surprisingly, those who had lost a twin in infancy or at birth sometimes mourned for life.

Some of the themes which emerged from the study echo those affecting surviving child twins. There was often guilt, for instance at not having been there to protect the twin, and there were sometimes feelings of inadequacy. Survivors felt that however much they achieved in life they could never be good enough for two.

Many adult lone twins had trouble relating to other people. Perhaps they were striving, and inevitably failing, to duplicate the closeness and intensity of the twin bond with someone else. Woodward found that some adult twins were intensely lonely, while others shunned closeness and described themselves as loners.

In 1989, with enthusiastic support from MBF, Joan Woodward founded the Lone Twin Network (LTN). (In the USA there is a Twinless Twins Support Group, founded by Raymond Brandt.) The Lone Twin Network has grown to several hundred members and offers support and contact to any lone twin over eighteen years old. Some get in touch soon after losing their twin, others many decades later – often after years of bottling up their emotions – by which time they have come to believe they must be weird to feel this way.

At whatever time lone twins hear of Lone Twin Network, there is often profound relief. Many are amazed to find that they are not alone in feeling bereaved, confused or lost themselves. Finally they can acknowledge the depth of their feelings.

The Lone Twin Network holds annual meetings for those who want to attend, and at some of these various other issues have been highlighted, such as the needs of parents of adult lone twins, and those of other siblings.

The impact of losing a twin in childhood resonates throughout life, but one is not always consciously aware of it.

Knowing that I can now make contact with other surviving twins who understand and have had a similar emotional reaction is very reassuring. My parents never spoke about my twin, who died suddenly aged five. I can understand that they must have been in a state of shock and denial for some considerable time and then found all the reminders too painful. The consequence is that I have no mementoes of my brother – just one photograph – and now both my parents are dead. I wonder if this is why I volunteered to create a Book of Remembrance for the Lone Twin Network.

What happens to the twinship is a fascinating if painful question. Because twins are so tightly linked, a lone twin may have difficulty in talking about 'I' instead of 'we'. Some survivors discover that their very identity appears to be under threat. For anyone who has recently been bereaved, catching a glimpse of the dead person out of the corner of one's eye is a common recurrent experience. In the case of a lone twin, looking in a mirror is often a long-term repeated reminder of the hurt. Being mistaken for one's identical twin by others can also be acutely painful.

Faith is a solace for some, especially those with a deep conviction that they will eventually be reunited with their twin, but, whatever their religious inclinations, most lone twins find it important to create some sort of memorial. It may be in the concrete sense of a plaque or headstone, or it could be by naming one of their own children after their twin.

For those whose twin was stillborn, obtaining the certificate can be a reassuring and tangible reminder of the co-twin's reality. Normally only parents are entitled to a stillbirth certificate, but as a result of MBF's efforts, an exception can be made so that the surviving twin is allowed to have a copy. All these things can help in dealing with the pain of no longer being a twin.

Chapter Fifteen

ADULT TWINS

Although people know very little about adult twins, they continue to find many of them fascinating. One pair who attract considerable curiosity is David and Frederick Barclay, identical twins now in their sixties. Together they built up an hotel empire from modest beginnings, buying up small properties, and their names are often in the financial pages of newspapers as a result of their successes: they recently bought the Ritz Hotel in London for £75 million. They own several newspapers and are amongst the wealthiest men in Britain (almost certainly the richest twins). However, what tends to capture public imagination most is the close and exclusive bond assumed to exist between them – they are very private and rarely inclined to grant interviews. Both having been married in the past, the brothers are believed still to wear matching pinstripe suits and live together in splendid seclusion on a Channel Island.

Two other highly successful twins were Norris and Ross McWhirter, who collaborated and thus excelled in many fields. After their degrees (and Blues for sprinting) at Oxford, they came to Fleet Street and were soon commissioned to compile the *Guinness Book of Records*, first published in 1955. Sadly Ross McWhirter was killed by an IRA bomb.

The Kray brothers were a particularly notorious set of twins, who came to fame for completely different reasons. At gangster Ronnie Kray's funeral in March 1995, the wreath of white chrysanthemums from his identical twin Reggie (younger by 45 minutes) spelt out the words: 'To the other half of me'. As Reggie said later, a part of him had died with Ronnie's death.

'I couldn't imagine living without my twin' is a common comment from twins. If twins cannot conceive of life without their twin, neither can singletons imagine what it might be like to have a twin. Psychologists are just beginning to appreciate that many adult twins have been affected in ways which more ordinary mortals barely understand.

Yet, despite the widespread popular appeal of adult twins, there has not been much systematic research into the subject. There is generally considered to be more to twins than just two people who happened to be born at the same time, but what exactly is it? An eerie psychic connection is often assumed to exist between twins – and sometimes there does indeed appear to be such a connection (a topic which is explored in several books including Peter Watson's *Twins*).

· *How Adult Twins See Themselves* ·

What are adult twins like? There can be no single answer to this question. Some twins are no closer than any two siblings, while a few identicals continue to have as adults an intense and exclusive relationship, living together, sharing a bedroom, choosing the same clothes and hairdos, working for the same company and finishing each other's sentences in conversations. Some pairs allocate daily tasks in such a way that only one will buy the newspaper, say, or post letters, and these can become chores that the other twin is unable to perform.

These are the exceptions who stand out. Many more do not.

Most adult twins seem to fall somewhere between these two extremes. On the whole, the closest links tend to be between identical twins, though it is not clear why. Is it purely because they are genetically the same, or because their parents brought them up as one unit on account of their striking physical similarity?

Twins with an antipathy to each other

The world at large expects twins to be somehow complementary to each other, yet for a few pairs, twinship is a constricting experience; it brings the serious disadvantages of being constantly compared and contrasted, and of having difficulty in asserting one's independence even as a young adult. This is especially prone to happen when one twin is dependent on the other and continually looks to his twin for guidance, something which can be unhealthy for both leader and led.

Reasons why some twins do not get on well include:

- constant fighting
- difficulty in developing their own identities; they may even be indistinguishable in family photographs
- extreme similarities, for example two intolerant people rarely get along
- feeling freakish: after all, the rest of the world is composed overwhelmingly of singletons
- unflattering comparisons: one twin can feel permanently inferior, as did the darker-skinned brother of a mixed-race pair; although he resented it, both boys seemed to take this for granted as the natural order, until they reached adulthood
- parental favouritism: the preferred one tends to blossom while his twin may feel he lives in his shadow.

Even when twins do not get on at all well, casual observers and acquaintances may assume they must, on account of their twinship, be best friends. This can be particularly hurtful – imagine being constantly mistaken for someone you cannot abide!

Occasionally, adult twins describe themselves as 'too close for comfort'. Some dislike the existence of another person who is so similar – after all, isn't there a common saying that we're all different? Twins may find it difficult to be together *because* they are uninhibited with each other, saying things they wouldn't dream of uttering to other people.

Some continue their rivalry into middle age and beyond, competing in terms of houses and their offspring's academic or sporting achievements. This can also happen with non-twins, though it tends to be more intense with same-sex twins. Sometimes the efforts are doomed to fail, as when one of the pair has a less well-paid job and simply cannot afford the same life-style as his twin.

Do many adult twins have problems? No, of course not. Most lead completely normal lives – and are no more or less balanced than any singleton, but one rarely hears about them. This is one of the difficulties of trying to find out what twins think of their twinship. As Dr Elizabeth Bryan says of twins of all ages who come to her clinic, 'I see the problems. People don't get in touch just to tell me that everything's all right.' So it is too with many kinds of research – those who respond tend to have a strong message to convey.

Being a twin is not an issue

A few pairs seem genuinely not to care either way about their twinship. It is no more and no less than the link between any two siblings. It is just there.

'I like him very much, and we are close,' says one woman of her fraternal twin brother, 'but no more close than to anyone else. In fact, I'd say I was closer to my older brother than to my twin.'

Being a twin is fun

Two identical twin girls, now both doctors, still seem to find great pleasure in their twinship, although one is the leader and the other follows. Their voices are especially alike and most people get them mixed up on the phone, though not in person. The younger one seems to find it less fun – she was always the follower.

We're still very close

Many twins find their twinship an enduring source of pleasure and support throughout life. The first person to hear of a twin's successes or failures is usually the co-twin, perhaps because they can be counted on to share the intensity of some of the joys and disappointments. One twin now facing redundancy in her forties finds her non-identical sister, although living in another country, particularly concerned and supportive.

· *Surveys of Twins* ·

Mary Rosambeau, a psychology graduate, social worker and mother of twins, has sought the views of hundreds of twins in their teens and beyond. Some of her findings are described in her book *How Twins Grow Up*. Amongst those who responded there was a high proportion of identical twins, so clearly these had something particular to say about their twinship, whereas non-identicals may have felt less strongly. This bias – or self-selection – amongst respondents means that percentages and figures are difficult to rely on, but Rosambeau's results are still fascinating.

Some of the advantages twins have mentioned in her book and elsewhere are:

- having someone close to you, a soul-mate as it were
- having a confidant, someone with whom you can be totally honest
- having someone who understands you, no matter what
- being special

- being popular socially (though twins may not be if they fight all the time!)
- protecting each other, presenting a united front whether at home, in the classroom or on the playing-field
- the practicalities: sharing chores, helping with homework
- someone to play tennis or board games with
- the benefits of competition (incidentally three female athletes who happen to be triplets recently gave this as one of the major reasons for their perseverance and success).

There are also disadvantages, according to the twins themselves, such as:

- society's ignorance: for instance, boy–girl pairs are often asked if they are identical (the mistake Shakespeare made with Viola and Sebastian is not unknown, even amongst Oxbridge dons)
- attracting attention for the wrong reasons: being valued purely for the twinship rather than as individuals, or being stared at as some kind of phenomenon
- being called 'the twins', or 'twinnie' – as one teenager told me, 'the worst thing was being summoned to the phone with the word "twinnies", even though only one of us was actually going to take the call.'
- unfair or insensitive comparisons, especially in such areas as physical appearance or exam results – 'She's the pretty one,' said one young woman. 'She always was. But I'm now the married one!'
- being responsible in some way for the other twin – for his feelings when he's left out, for his safety when playing together
- being too dependent on each other
- material disadvantages
- lack of parental time and attention.

Interestingly, the issues adult twins consider important are much the same as the ones focused on in this book from the child-rearing point of view. Some of them can be altered for the better. Although one may not be able to do much about society's ignorance and preconceptions, today's parent is in a good position to be aware of the problems their twins face and to help them get the most from being twins.

· *The Opposite Sex* ·

Any outsider can find it hard to become involved in a twin's social life, and this affects many emotional and romantic relationships. It is difficult to intrude on the closeness of twins and, whether or not the twins are of the same sex, prospective partners may feel that they need to obtain permission from the other twin before a relationship can become serious. Twin (and triplet) girls often say that any boyfriend has to get on well with all of them. The thought of such a vetting procedure can put off many interested males.

René Zazzo believed that twins often marry later than singletons and found that many did not marry at all, perhaps out of a sense of loyalty to the twinship. Therapist Audrey Sandbank points out that expectations regarding marriage can be very high. In fact, many of us, whether twins or singletons, have excessively high expectations of our marriages and partnerships, but in twins it may be particularly unrealistic to assume that any bond as deep as that of twinship can be developed.

There is anecdotal evidence that the continuing intimate relationship between twins can make the spouses of twins feel excluded or insecure. As one woman says:

> I actually introduced my twin brother to his future wife, who
> was a close colleague of mine. Yet for many years into their

marriage it was clear that my sister-in-law was very jealous
of me. And it is not as if my brother and I were ever insepa-
rable.

This probably says more about the sister-in-law's assumptions about twins' relationships than it does about these
twins.

When only one twin marries or develops a lasting
relationship, trouble can result, with the other feeling acutely
left out or on the shelf. It can cause estrangement between
the twins. Often the unhappiness is temporary, and in due
course the single twin finds his feet and makes his own way.
Occasionally the remaining twin hastily finds a partner too
and it may be someone unsuitable: a distress purchase, as it
were.

On the other hand, the twin left behind is sometimes
relieved rather than upset at remaining single:

> After all, the marriage and moving away of one of the pair
> also eliminates some of the disadvantages of twinship, which
> can be a liberating experience.

Occasionally there are other unusual facets of twins' relationships with others:

- Young adult twins may play tricks on girlfriends or
  boyfriends. As one nineteen-year-old says:

> When I was seeing someone I actually didn't like very much,
> I sent my identical brother once to meet her in my place. She
> didn't crack it, although she might have done in time. He
> didn't like her either, as it happens, but he thought it was a
> lark playing this massive trick on her!

- Twins sometimes marry other twins. Exactly why this
  should happen is not clear, but we do tend to choose as
  partners people like ourselves.

- Twins, usually same-sex pairs, may be attracted to the same person. In fact, this seems to happen far less often than one would suppose and possibly slightly less often than it occurs with any singleton siblings. Many twins say they would never find the same person attractive because they have different tastes, but it also could be a manifestation of an unspoken taboo, as in the case of incest.

- A few people enter into bigamous relationships with both members of a twin pair simultaneously. At university one undergraduate alternately bedded two identical sisters for several months, a situation one of them knew about and accepted, while the other one (who happened to be the dominant one of the twinship) was apparently unaware of events. And at least one woman is known to co-habit with identical brothers, all three of them sharing a bedroom and a relationship. When she appeared on television with this story, it was clear that she treated the men as one unit. How serious are such relationships? It is impossible for outsiders to know.

· *Did the Parents of Adult Twins* · *Get It Right?*

This question is very relevant to today's parents of multiples. Again, there is no one answer, and no formal research has been carried out into the subject. It seems fair to generalize from the wealth of anecdotes and observations available that those twins who were helped from an early age to be individuals do best as independent adults. For example:

> I felt that my mother, who was a single parent for much of our childhood, coped very well indeed and had a lot of

insight too. She cultivated us as individuals, so that we each grew up to have a sense of our own worth. And I am very grateful for it, because it couldn't have been easy.

Several psychotherapists have found that it sometimes becomes evident in adulthood that things might have worked out better if parents had done things differently:

> Mine could frankly have done better. I thought our upbringing was normal at the time, but looking back I think my parents were so tickled by having identical twins that they failed to see we needed to develop away from each other as well as from them. We were treated more like Siamese twins. And I think we were treated as babies for far longer than if we'd been single-born because we were so cute.

All is not necessarily lost, however. Adult twins who are unable to function well independently may still be helped. Joining TAMBA's Adult Twins Group can help adult twins find their own way and gain control of their own lives as individuals for the first time.

What are today's children likely to think?

Thirty years ago there was little awareness of the needs of twins and higher multiples, so perhaps it shouldn't be surprising that a few have had enduring problems in adulthood. But things have changed. There are more multiples born, for a start. Medical care has advanced, parenting has become less rigid, and information has never been as accessible as it is today. Taking into account the research now being done into the issues concerning multiples, it may well be that today's youngsters will fare better – psychologically as well as medically – than they would have a couple of decades ago. However, it would be wrong to be complacent about the challenges families face. Audrey Sandbank points out that the twin problems she sees in family therapy are much the same as the ones she dealt with twenty years ago.

Advice from adult twins

Happily, few of the adult twins I have spoken to are particularly critical of their own parents, but several wanted to pass on advice to parents of young twins. Since the points they make also appear under different headings elsewhere in this book, I apologize for the obvious repetition, but the issues raised do seem to be important recurring themes.

- Don't dress them alike, or at least only as small babies.
- Give them separate bedrooms as soon as you can – and as soon as they want them.
- Be fair where possible.
- Avoid insensitive (and often pointless) comparisons.
- Help them function separately at school as well as at home.
- Give them the freedom to be themselves.

This last comment is echoed by therapist Audrey Sandbank, who believes that twins should be given choices as they grow up, so that they can make up their own minds about being close or apart.

· *Twin Phenomena and Twin Studies* ·

Infant twins put up for adoption are no longer placed with separate families if it can possibly be helped, but at one time they were, often without any of the parties involved being told that twins had even been born. This practice resulted in a number of twins being reared apart, sometimes in very different households and without knowing for many years that they had a twin somewhere. In some cases the twins discovered their twinship in adulthood (some suspected it earlier) and made efforts to be reunited with their co-twin.

There have been some eerie results. The so-called 'Jim twins' from Ohio, USA, are among the best-known examples of amazing coincidental similarities between twins reared apart. Adopted separately in 1939, both were given the forename James by their adoptive families. This is unremarkable, but there were some surprising parallels between them. When they met up around the age of 40, the two Jims found that they both had sons with the same names; they had each married a woman called Linda and later divorced, each to marry a Betty; they had several habits in common, including common ones like nail-biting and more unusual ones like leaving love-notes around the house; they drank the same type of beer, smoked the same brand of cigarettes, had the same hobbies and sporting interests, and suffered from much the same ailments.

For many years psychologists from the University of Minnesota have been studying twins, including those brought up separately. In 1983 Professor Thomas Bouchard Jr established the Minnesota Center for Twin and Adoption Research. It has several aims and functions: some are educational, while others include helping those still trying to find their co-twin. The Center is based in Minneapolis, which is in itself interesting Minneapolis and the adjoining town of St Paul have long been known as the Twin Cities for geographical reasons, though it is St Paul which is considered to be the state capital of Minnesota.

Twins reared apart allow scientists to gain useful insights into the relative importance of nature and nurture, and also raise questions about the possibility of extra-sensory perception (ESP) or psychic communication. The Minnesota Study of Twins Reared Apart is just one of the Center's projects. In this programme, adult twins are invited to the university for a week of in-depth assessment to elucidate the environmental and genetic factors responsible for various medical and psychological characteristics.

Some of the similarities found when twins meet up have been striking, as in the case of the Jim twins, but a few could be simply coincidental. What, for instance, is the probability of two unrelated people wearing similar coats on a cold day? Clearly there is a likelihood that they might just have chosen the same coat by chance, especially if it is of a type widely available. If you buy clothes at Marks & Spencer, for instance, you won't necessarily have to go far to find someone else – probably of similar age to yourself – wearing the same garment.

It could be that when twins show these similarities they are pounced upon and considered significant, but the rest of the time such coincidences might be conveniently ignored because they are not interesting enough. This topic is outside the scope of this book, but it has been nicely covered in Peter Watson's *Twins*, where you can find out more about the Jim and other reunited twins, as well as other popular aspects of Professor Bouchard's work.

There are many other twin registers around the world and they all focus on different areas of study. The Louisville Twin Study in Kentucky is a long-term project into growth and mental development which began some 30 years ago and is widely quoted. Then there is the Institute of Psychiatry register of adult twins in London, which was set up in 1969 and which, it is hoped, will answer some important questions on mental health.

The twins database at St Thomas's Hospital, London, holds information on over 1200 twins and is expanding fast. Recently Gemini, the world's first medical research company based entirely on twin studies, was set up jointly by Australian and British doctors, including the St Thomas's group. One of the research interests is osteoporosis (brittle bones) which affects one in three women and around one in 12 men. Another is osteoarthritis (degenerative joint dis-ease).

Rheumatologists at St Thomas's are hoping to clarify to what extent osteoarthritis is due to genetics and to what extent it is due to environment (for instance, plain old wear and tear). Identical twins are genetically indistinguishable, so any differences between them are caused by environmental factors. This is a fascinating and potentially useful project, to which twins can contribute if they are interested. Not surprisingly a huge number of adult twins, both identical and fraternal, have so far volunteered to help in this and other research.

It is only fair to point out that the classic 'twin study' method described does have some pitfalls:

- Even if two people have the same genes, the genes will not necessarily be expressed in exactly the same way. A gene can, in effect, lie dormant or be inactive. We know this happens with the X chromosome, for instance.

- Being brought up together or living together for a long time makes people similar in many ways – both physically and psychologically – so that some similarities between identical twins reared together may be due to their shared environment. If this factor is ignored, one could over-estimate the important of genetics.

- Some diseases, like diabetes or high blood pressure, are influenced by poor growth in the womb. Therefore, if (or when) these conditions seem commoner in some pairs of twins, they may not be genetically based – the pre-birth environment could be to blame instead.

These are all factors that have to be taken into account. They do not invalidate any of the research and I would not wish to detract in any way from the important work now in progress, or from future research as yet undreamt of, that could shed light not only on twins but on life itself.

APPENDIX

· *Chorionicity* ·

One of the newest and perhaps most promising applications of ultrasound is in detecting what is known as chorionicity: whether twins in the womb are separated by two chorionic membranes or just one. Most twins have two and are called dichorionic, while a minority will be monochorionic.

There is a subtle difference between zygosity (identicalness) and chorionicity, even though, according to a recent survey, not all obstetricians realize it! All non-identicals (DZ) and about one-third of identicals (MZ) are dichorionic, leaving the remaining identicals (MZ) as monochorionic.

Whether identicals turn out to be monochorionic or dichorionic depends on when the fertilized ovum splits into two:

- If it happens within three days of fertilization, the twins are dichorionic.
- If the ovum splits after three days, the twins are monochorionic.

How can one tell?

When the twins are dichorionic, a small wedge-shaped area (called the lambda sign) is visible between the two sacs on scans between ten and fourteen weeks of pregnancy. It's sometimes seen a bit later on too, but not reliably.

What's the point?

Many of the twin pregnancies which come to grief are mono-chorionic (twin-to-twin transfusion syndrome (see below) being the main cause of death. If there is only one chorion, it may be advisable to monitor the pregnancy more closely, with scans every two weeks until, at least 24 weeks. Meanwhile, the majority of women – those with a dichorionic twin pregnancy – can be reassured that they fall into a low-risk group. Many teaching hospitals now assess chorionicity, but it isn't routine everywhere.

Are your twins monochorionic?

Unless your hospital assesses chorionicity, you may not be sure, but your twin pregnancy is definitely dichorionic – and therefore relatively low-risk – if either:

- the placentas are separate, or
- you have a boy–girl pair.

· Twin-to-Twin Transfusion Syndrome · (TTS)

This is a rare but dangerous complication of some identical (MZ) twin pregnancies. It affects those which have only one chorion (see above).

In TTS, there is only one placenta, with blood vessels that interconnect the fetuses, so that they share their blood flow unequally. Blood is shunted from one baby to the other; it's effectively a blood transfusion (hence the name of the condition). TTS often works out badly for both babies.

What can happen?

The so-called donor ends up receiving much less blood than

his twin. As the pregnancy continues, he becomes much smaller, anaemic, possibly shrivelled and may have brain damage.

Meanwhile, the recipient, who gets more of the blood, is larger and redder. He may have heart failure and will usually produce more amniotic fluid, resulting in hydramnios. In fact a woman's discomfort from hydramnios is often the first sign that something is amiss. (For more on hydramnios, see Chapter 2.)

That is what happens in full-blown TTS. Happily, many babies are affected to a much lesser extent and may just show some discrepancy in size or colouring. It is said that the biblical twins Jacob and Esau may have had TTS, which would explain why Jacob was so pale and Esau so red.

It is likely that around 15 per cent of monochorionic pregnancies overall – or about one in every 30 twin pregnancies – are affected by TTS to some degree because of their blood vessel interconnections.

Making the diagnosis

If your twins are monochorionic, the pregnancy can be monitored regularly by USS for signs of TTS. But what if you don't know the chorionicity, perhaps because your hospital doesn't yet look for this? If there are two placentas, or the babies are of different sexes, don't worry – they're dichorionic and won't get TTS.

If you still don't know the chorionicity, don't panic, but look out for early symptoms like discomfort or a rapidly expanding belly. Get your doctor or midwife to take any symptoms of this sort seriously, to prevent the consequences of severe untreated TTS. Make a fuss if you have to. TTS is still rare and there may be one or two professionals who know little about this condition. You would not easily forgive them – or yourself – if you lost your twins because you didn't get the right attention in time.

Treatment

Unfortunately, severe TTS can be fatal for the babies, but there are now two promising new ways of treating it. Both are still at the stage of being evaluated. They are not widely available and are being used only in selected pregnancies badly affected by TTS. The main methods are:

- Amniodrainage, which involves drawing off quantities of amniotic fluid by amniocentesis at about weekly intervals. This treats the effect of TTS rather than its cause.

- Laser treatment of the interconnecting blood vessels, which can coagulate the cross-channels. It is done using a fine laser probe between 15 and 28 weeks of pregnancy.

Both types of treatment are carried out under local anaesthetic and your partner can usually be present. It's early days yet, but so far laser therapy seems to have the edge. Several hundred treatments have been done at centres worldwide, notably at the Harris Birthright Centre in London. It seems that even in severe cases laser treatment can give a 70 per cent chance of at least one healthy baby and a 50 per cent chance of two healthy babies. The babies also appear to be healthier than after treatment with amniodrainage.

· Selective Termination ·

Also known as selective birth or selective feticide, this refers to selectively terminating the life of one fetus of a twin (or triplet) pregnancy, while leaving the remaining one(s) intact.

Although it has been done since the late 1970s for a variety of serious disorders, selective termination is not something the average couple knows about. In fact, the first time most people are likely to hear of it is when one of their babies is diagnosed as having a severe or even lethal malformation.

This in itself is an extremely distressing discovery to make at a highly emotional time. Taking in new facts and figures is particularly hard at such moments and yet before long the couple will have to make a major decision based on what they understand and how they feel about the situation.

In a twin pregnancy where only one baby is found to have an abnormality, the choice is really three-way:

1 The pregnancy can continue without intervention, in the knowledge that one baby may be born severely disabled. In some cases, the healthy baby may even be put at risk from continuing to share a womb with his twin, not because the condition is in any way catching, but because the diseased baby may have a mechanical effect. This can happen especially in cases of anencephaly (a very severe skull malformation).

2 The entire pregnancy can be terminated, with the loss of a presumed healthy baby along with the sick one.

3 The pregnancy can be selectively terminated. (For those of you who want technical details, see the section below entitled 'The procedure itself'.)

The decision

Guided by your specialist, you and your partner have to decide together on the right course of action in the light of the exact diagnosis. A baby who is unlikely to live long after birth may be agonizing to bear, but poses different problems from the baby who grows up in constant pain or who becomes a heavy burden to his parents, and to his twin, perhaps for decades. Ask your doctor as many questions as you need to, and jot down the answers so you can remember them later.

Your own religious beliefs and family situation, including

commitments to any children you have already, also come into the equation. The doctor cannot decide for you, but can provide the information you need and perhaps also act as a sounding-board for your thoughts. Your doctor's own beliefs should not influence your decision. Should your doctor object on principle to selective (or any other) termination, you are entitled to be referred without delay to someone else.

Close family and friends may be very supportive, but they don't always understand the mixed feelings which are natural in this situation. It's hard for some people to grasp that anyone left with one surviving baby (which is all most pregnancies produce, after all) could be hankering for anything more. If you want, your specialist or the MBF can probably put you in touch with another couple who have gone through this experience.

The procedure itself

Selective termination is carried out between 18 and 22 weeks of pregnancy. The main time constraint against acting earlier is that the abnormality probably won't have been picked up before 18 weeks.

First, an ultrasound has to establish that the fetuses each have their own placental circulation. If they are monochorionic (see page 319) they will share a blood flow and selective termination can't be done because of the high risk of both babies dying as a result.

Assuming the fetuses are dichorionic, scanning is then used to locate the abnormal fetus and his placenta. Under ultrasound control, a fine needle is carefully passed through the woman's abdomen and into the affected baby. An injection of local anaesthetic is given; this is 100 per cent successful and works immediately.

The remaining baby is then checked just to make sure he's still well. If you are rhesus negative, you will need an injection of anti-D at this stage to prevent complications of rhesus incompatibility, exactly as if you had just miscarried, had a complete termination or indeed delivered a baby.

Immediately afterwards, you may lose the sensation of kicking from that part of your belly. Over the next few weeks, the dead fetus shrinks to a large extent, though there will usually be some evidence of it at delivery.

What about the other baby? There is believed to be a miscarriage rate of 5 to 10 per cent for the survivor. The later the procedure is done, the greater the risk seems to be, so you'll have frequent scans to monitor the remainder of your pregnancy.

More than fifteen years' experience of selective termination in centres all over the world suggests that the presence of the dead fetus alongside the survivor causes few physical problems. In fact, the situation seems to resemble the many cases where nature causes one baby of a multiple pregnancy to perish before birth. Premature labour appears to be a risk, but this is a hazard of twin pregnancy anyway, and it's not clear that the risk is significantly greater after selective termination.

Emotions

It is entirely normal to feel sad and to grieve for your lost baby – even for your lost role as a parent of twins. Your reaction may not be obvious right away. For example, it may not be until your healthy surviving baby is born that you fully appreciate your bereavement. By then other people, including some midwives and doctors, may consider that you should somehow have 'got over it' and be concentrating on looking after your live baby. They do not mean to be thoughtless, but that's how it can come across.

You may indeed be able to put your loss behind you, but this isn't possible for everyone. Unresolved grief can make it an uphill struggle to go on with normal life and especially with caring for a baby who should, had all been well, have had a healthy companion born alongside him.

It may help you, as it has others, to acknowledge in tangible ways your lost baby as an individual:

- Perhaps you'll want to see him at the time of delivery. If so, ask in advance. Staff may just assume that you don't.

- You may later want to have a photo of the fetus, or perhaps a painting or a copy of an ultrasound picture. If you don't want to see your dead baby at delivery, you may still want someone to take a photo, just in case.

- Giving your dead baby a name will help identify him and could help you and your partner talk about him more easily. Remember that, as with two live-born twins, it may be kinder on your surviving baby not to have a matching name.

- A funeral or memorial service can be arranged if you wish.

- Counselling may help you and your partner come to terms with what happened. Contact your GP, SATFA or MBF if you would like support, or get in touch with TAMBA Bereavement Support Group.

Before long, you will need to tell your surviving child about his co-twin. The long-term emotional effects of selective termination on a survivor aren't yet known, but it's probably best to be open with the rest of the family. Things have a habit of coming out and you wouldn't want him to find out from someone else. Even without being told of their twinship, surviving lone twins can somehow be acutely aware that they had a companion before birth (there's more on this subject in Chapter 14).

You need not of course give a young child a detailed account of how his twin died – merely the information that he was very sick and didn't live long enough to be born. This requires a great deal of sensitivity. The survivor may need reassurance that he was not to blame in any way for what happened.

· *Embryo Reduction in Higher-Order* · *Multiple Pregnancies*

This is also called multifetal pregnancy reduction. In this procedure, a triplet, quadruplet, or even higher-order pregnancy is reduced to a twin (or even singleton) pregnancy to reduce the risk of disability and thus increase the chances of producing a healthy baby. (The technique is described below under 'The procedure itself' for those who want to know the details.)

There are many ethical considerations and you won't want to contemplate embryo reduction at all if you have conscientious objections to termination. Even among doctors who themselves practise termination there are different shades of opinion. Some obstetricians believe there can never be any justification for reducing a pregnancy which is progressing well, no matter how many embryos there are. However, as I said earlier in the book, one at a time is the normal way for humans to reproduce. One or two specialists consider that reducing triplet pregnancies to twins (or even to singletons) is perfectly rational and justifiable since multiples, including twins, tend to fare less well than single babies.

Both of these are extreme views. Most obstetricians probably fall somewhere between the two, especially since the outlook for twins and triplets is improving. They would be prepared to reduce a quad, quin or sextuplet pregnancy on the basis that carrying fewer embryos can increase the 'take-home' baby rate.

The decision

Only you and your partner can decide what's right for your circumstances and the limitations of your resources – social, emotional and financial – and you have to decide without the benefit of hindsight. It is a gamble. If you do nothing, you could end up with a number of beautiful healthy babies, or you could lose some or all. Quads and more do face a higher risk of death or disability, mainly because the babies are more likely to be both small and premature.

The procedure itself

If you go ahead, embryo reduction is done at about twelve weeks or more. This applies even if you were having treatment for infertility, and hence frequent scans from early on, which told you long before twelve weeks how many embryos you were carrying. It's worth waiting a little before embryo reduction not only to give yourselves time to decide, but because there is some risk of natural embryo loss before twelve weeks.

The choice as to which embryos to terminate is generally made on technical grounds, depending on which are most accessible. Otherwise the principles are much the same as for selective termination, described earlier in this Appendix.

Guided by ultrasound, a needle is passed through the woman's abdomen and into the embryo's chest and local anaesthetic is then injected. This works immediately. If many embryos are to be terminated, the procedure is sometimes done in two stages a week or so apart. Embryo reduction can also be done through the woman's cervix, but this is less common.

Technically, the success rate approaches 100 per cent and complications are unusual. Frequent scans are done to keep an eye on progress for the rest of the pregnancy. There seem to be few physical side-effects apart from a risk of miscarriage, but, as research suggests, this is no greater than the miscarriage risk in most multiple pregnancies.

Because the procedure is done early on in a pregnancy, there is less to see at delivery than with selective termination.

Emotions

An element of sadness or even guilt, no matter how unfounded, may tinge the rest of your pregnancy. You and your partner may feel uneasy at having terminated one or more embryos, especially as the 'choice' as to which survived has to be made more or less arbitrarily. It may help you to talk things over, perhaps with a counsellor. You can discuss this with TAMBA, MBF or your GP.

Many pregnancies of triplets and more result from assisted-reproduction techniques, a fact which saddens and angers some parents and their doctors. It would obviously be better to have avoided these very high-order pregnancies in the first place, for instance by closer monitoring of the effects of fertility treatments. In undergoing embryo reduction, however, you may substantially increase your chance of achieving your aim: having at least one healthy baby of your own. Psychological research from the USA suggests that 96 per cent of families who opted for embryo reduction would make the same decision again.

· *Basic Equipment for Newborns* ·

If you've already had one baby, you have some idea of what equipment is available – and what is actually needed, which is not the same thing. With multiples, you will obviously need some different items of equipment and may have less disposable cash. There will also be less time for some of the niceties, such as bootees, mittens and pram shoes.

Clothing

You will need at least:

vests: two for each baby
stretch suits: three each
jackets: two each
bonnets: one each (for winter, or if the babies are very small)
blankets: one each
cot sheets: two each

This really is the bare minimum. The more you have of these items, the easier life will be. Make sure all the clothing is machine-washable.

Other useful items are *shawls* (one each) and several '*dribble cloths*' each (you can use terry nappies or muslin squares). These also come into their own to protect a sheet or blanket.

Equipment

Baby bath (preferably with stand)
Nappy-changing bag or mat (preferably both)
Baby listener (can be very useful)

Cot: you can often manage with just one for six weeks or more, depending on the size of your twins. They can sleep end to end – this way they may kick each other but are less likely to scratch each other's faces. Or they can sleep side by side – the advantage here is that the babies can both be positioned near the foot of the cot and the bedclothes arranged to come up no higher than their shoulders (this is thought to be an important factor in preventing cot death). To save confusion at night, it is helpful to keep each baby in the same place, e.g. Daniel on the right and Sam on the left.

Car seat for each baby, if you have a car. Rear-facing baby seats are ideal for the very young. They usually have a handle so they can be removed easily and carried like a basket, even when a baby's asleep in one. In the house, the car seat can double as reclining chair and may save you buying bouncing cradles (you would otherwise need one of these for each baby). Don't put a baby seat in the front of the car if you have a passenger airbag: in an emergency, this inflates forcefully and could break a baby's neck.

Baby slings: useful if you and your partner intend to carry a baby each, but potentially damaging to your back if you are planning to carry two babies at a time yourself. It may be the only way you can get on a bus unaided, for instance, but your twins will soon get heavy, and what seemed like a reasonable weight when you left the house can become unbearable fifteen minutes later.

Pram: you will need one if you go out on foot. For a short while you can often manage with a single pram, if you already have one, but soon your babies will be too big. A big twin pram can last you a long time but has the drawback that it may not fit into the car. An alternative is a double buggy – some types with bucket seats are suitable for the very young – but it may not be up to the job once your babies become toddlers and, while they're still small, a buggy gives less protection than a pram against the elements.

Buying second-hand often works out well with equipment for twins and more, and local twins' clubs often have used equipment on offer. If you buy things in this way, or borrow equipment from friends, make sure everything's safe and in good clean condition. In the case of a cot, for instance, you may want to buy a new mattress. A good twin pram bought second-hand usually still has some resale value when you've finished with it. Second-hand clothes are often harsh to the touch, but can be all right.

The good news? You do not need:

- nightdresses for the babies
- cot bumpers (they look nice, but a baby can get trapped inside one and later a more mobile infant can climb on to it and fall out of the cot)
- cot pillows (because of the risk of suffocation)
- special pram sheets (fold a cot sheet instead)
- baby changing unit (a changing mat on a chest of drawers is more useful. The mat also has sides which will help prevent the baby rolling off the chest of drawers to some extent. This is a common accident risk because the mother's attention may be distracted by the other twin.)
- Moses baskets or cribs (they are soon outgrown and, as you would have bought two, doubly extravagant).

· *Cot Death (Sudden Infant Death* · *Syndrome)*

Cot death (SIDS) is rare, but it is slightly more common in twins and multiple births, especially those who are premature or low in birth weight. It is worth knowing about cot death and what you can do to reduce the risk. Nevertheless, the vast majority of small babies survive the first year without mishap, so try not to worry too much.

Cot death affects babies under a year old and mostly under

six months. Although nobody really knows the cause, overheating and overwhelming infection – to which new babies lack immunity – are thought to be important. Recent research has highlighted measures to prevent some cot death and these seem to be working. In the UK, SIDS has become far less common following a government campaign giving advice to parents on the sleeping position of young babies and other matters.

What you can do

- Always place your babies on their backs to sleep unless your doctor has given you a specific reason not to. The side will do too, though a baby may roll on to his front unless you extend the underneath arm. Don't use wedges or rolled up towels. Make sure the babies' heads cannot get completely covered by bedclothes.

- Don't smoke, either during or after pregnancy. Keep your babies out of smoky atmospheres and ask visitors not to smoke in the house.

- Don't let your babies become overheated. The ideal room temperature is around 65°F (18°C). Buy a room thermometer if necessary. Unless the weather is exceptionally cold, central heating can usually be turned off at night.

- Never overdress your babies, especially if they're ill or running a fever. Avoid sheepskins, hot-water bottles and electric blankets altogether.

- Don't let very young babies get too cold, either. They need to be wrapped up outside in cold weather.

- In some countries such as New Zealand, cot-death campaigns have advocated breast-feeding as a preventive measure. It may help protect against cot death, but there is no proof of this.

- If you suspect one of your babies is unwell, get medical advice.

Parents sometimes ask about apnoea alarms, which are designed to go off if a baby stops breathing momentarily. Current medical opinion is that these alarms are not in themselves enough to save lives that might have been lost to cot death. They can give false alarms or, on occasion, fail to sound and give a false sense of reassurance. Although apnoea alarms can be helpful, they should not be used without medical supervision.

You should phone 999 or go straight to hospital (accident and emergency department) if a baby

- stops breathing
- turns blue
- is very drowsy or unrousable.

After a cot death

If there has been a cot death in your family, you will no doubt worry about whether it could happen to the surviving twin. It is vital to keep a very close watch on the other baby, so he will almost certainly be taken into hospital immediately for a few days' observation to prevent a further tragedy.

There is also a slightly higher risk of cot death in any baby you have later. In the UK, a programme called CONI (Care of the Next Infant) provides support for the subsequent baby and can help identify those at extra-high risk.

Cot death is rare but is without doubt a devastating experience. As a parent, you will want to know why it happened, but it is not always possible to give an answer. Although it is understandable that you may want to go through and analyse your baby's last few days and hours, try not to blame yourself.

In the case of twins or more, there are also other complex issues surrounding infant death (see Chapter 14). You can get help from TAMBA Bereavement Support Group, MBF

Bereavement Clinics, and the Foundation for the Study of Infant Deaths (addresses on page 345).

· *Attention Deficit Disorder* ·

Attention deficit disorder (ADD) is also known as hyperactivity or, more accurately, attention deficit hyperactivity disorder (ADHD), the term officially recognized by the American Psychiatric Association.

ADHD probably exists all over the world, but its diagnosis is much more readily accepted in the USA and Australia. It may be overdiagnosed in some countries but it is probably underdiagnosed here. In the UK, ADHD tends to be put in the same category as dyslexia, ME (myalgic encephalomyelitis; also known as chronic fatigue syndrome) and food allergies: all conditions which are hard to prove and sometimes thought to be the product of overactive middle-class imaginations. Hence children with ADHD can miss out on treatment.

Who has it?

ADHD is thought to affect between 2 and 10 per cent of all children, depending on whether or not one counts mild cases. Boys usually outnumber girls by a factor of three to one. Genetics are important – a sibling of someone with ADHD has a 30 to 40 per cent chance of being affected too, while if one identical twin has it, the other will also have it in 90 per cent of cases. Twins have a particularly high incidence anyway. Professor David Hay from Australia found ADHD to be nearly twice as common in twins as in singletons. The twin–singleton difference existed in both sexes, but ADHD was more common in boys, with up to 16 per cent of twin boys having the condition. Twins with reading problems tended to have more ADHD symptoms in this study. Why ADHD is more common in twins is not known, and research continues. ADHD can run in families from one generation to the next. Grandma may point out that a small child is 'just like his Dad was as a youngster'.

Symptoms

Typical symptoms are:

- lack of attention and concentration
- overactivity, with constant fidgeting
- disorganization
- lack of social skills
- clumsiness
- disruptive behaviour.

In mild cases, ADHD can be difficult to define: all young children show these characteristics to some extent. You would not, for instance, expect a five-year-old to be as organized as an adult, nor to be able to concentrate for as long as a university student. Twins seem to have particularly poor powers of concentration, but this may be just because they interrupt and divert each other.

Usually, symptoms of ADHD come to light in toddlerhood or the pre-school years, or else early on in primary school. Occasionally babies who are very active in the womb later turn out to have ADHD.

ADHD can seriously interfere with learning and behaviour and lead to long-term underachievement. Because children with ADHD cannot concentrate for long and tend to make silly careless mistakes, they may do badly at school. Some children with ADHD do well except in certain types of work, like project work, which require a high degree of organization and tidiness.

Most are not 'stupid' at all, but their behaviour can be

ridiculed at times. Because they may have difficulty making friends, they may lack self-esteem.

However, a few children with ADHD have added difficulties with language (for example, with speech, understanding long instructions or answering open-ended questions). There is also a connection in some cases between ADHD and dyslexia, which may make schoolwork all the more challenging.

Symptoms often improve in the teens, but by then low self-esteem and poor work at school may have already left their mark.

Making the diagnosis

Sometimes the diagnosis is very obvious, or perhaps someone like your GP, health visitor or teacher has suggested it as a possibility. Consulting a paediatrician, child psychiatrist or educational psychologist will usually tell you whether your children have ADHD.

Clinching the diagnosis is a matter of talking to parents and observing children, supplemented, perhaps, by special questionnaires. There's no laboratory test for ADHD. Special scans of the brain are known to show subtle abnormalities, but these are used only in research and it is not yet feasible to scan on a large scale.

It is important to diagnose ADHD when it exists, but also not to diagnose it when the real difficulty lies elsewhere, for instance when a family breaks up, a co-twin has special needs, there is a bereavement or a child is being bullied at school. Just to complicate matters, ADHD can of course co-exist with any of these other problems too.

What is the cause?

Nobody knows the exact cause of ADHD but one thing is certain: it is not the parents' fault. Children don't develop the condition because they weren't disciplined enough or because they ate the wrong foods. At the moment it seems that children with ADHD are just made that way – perhaps the levels of chemicals that transmit messages in the brain (so-called neuro-transmitters) are subtly different from other children's, but this is only speculation.

Coping with ADHD

After the condition has been diagnosed, the most important step is to accept it, but it is not always easy to love a child just as he is, especially if he's different from his siblings. Youngsters with ADHD can be very difficult and may have few friends, so their family may be the only source of good feelings. It is important to be loving yet firm in handling and to set clear limits and regular routines. This may not be enough to solve the problem, but it helps.

Diet is a factor in some cases. Here the blame may lie with one or a few foods, such as some artificial colourings, and taking them out of the diet sometimes helps. In a few cases, a more restricted diet may be useful. However, it is important to be careful with this approach. Putting a growing child on a restricted diet can do more harm than good. Diets which eliminate more than just the odd item are best given under the supervision of a dietitian. Ask your doctor.

Some drugs work well for many children with ADHD. These medicines are, paradoxically, stimulant drugs like methylphenidate (Ritalin) and dexamphetamine. When they work, their effect can be astonishing, but they do need to be given regularly. They suppress symptoms rather than cure the condition. Most importantly, they need to be given under the supervision of a specialist.

You can get more information from the Hyperactive Children's Support Group (address on page 344).

· *A Framework Policy for Schools* ·

Headteacher Pat Preedy, together with TAMBA, has formulated this policy to help schools consider and meet the needs of twins and higher multiples.

Introduction

Before their children start at a nursery or school, parents should be consulted about their development and needs and how to introduce them to school. During the children's time at school, parents and staff need to review their progress and the educational provision. It may be difficult for parents to help both children with their learning (hearing both read during the same evening, for example). Arrangements such as hearing each child read on alternate nights may have to be made.

Individuality

Twins and higher-order multiples have their own personalities and emotional needs. Adults and children need to be able to identify individuals and to call them by name. They should be respected as individuals and never referred to as 'the twins' or 'the triplets', etc.

- Reward each child as an individual.
- Never compare children to their detriment.
- Do not label the children, e.g. 'the clever one', 'the naughty one'.
- Arrange separate parents' evenings and discuss the children's progress at separate times.
- Where applicable, give each child a separate letter to take home and expect each child to bring individual replies, money, etc., from home.

- Be aware that the children and parents will compare progress whether they are in the same class or not. It is important that one child does not lose confidence, particularly with reading.

Separation/keeping together

Putting twins and higher-order multiples into separate classes requires careful consideration and consultation with parents and the children themselves. Some children may never have been separated.

A flexible approach is required and an understanding of the fact that children may have a double separation to cope with when they start school: from parents and from their twin.

When twins and higher multiples are separated it is frequently the dominant child who becomes insecure and the other child who blossoms.

If twins and higher multiples are together they have no privacy and have to share in telling what happened at school.

Be positive

Twins and higher-order multiples enjoy a special relationship. They have had to learn to share and take turns. They are frequently more independent and good at dressing/undressing. They are special and people give them special attention.

With understanding and support where necessary, twins and higher multiples develop as individuals with their own strengths while enjoying and celebrating the fact that they are multiples.

FURTHER READING

Ainslie, Ricardo C., *The Psychology of Twinship*, University of Nebraska Press (Nebraska) 1995

Australian MBA Inc & Department of Psychology, La Trobe University, *La Trobe Study – Twins in School*, La Trobe University (Melbourne) 1991

Botting, B.J., Macfarlane, A.J., Price, F.V. (eds), *Three, Four and More: National Study of Triplet and Higher Order Births*, HMSO (London) 1990

Bryan, Elizabeth, *Twins and Higher Multiple Births: A Guide to Their Nature and Nurture*, Edward Arnold (London) 1992.

Bryan, Elizabeth, *Twins, Triplets and More: Their nature, development, and care*, MBF (London) 1995

Buckler, John, *The Adolescent Years: The ups and downs of growing up*, Castlemead Publications (Ware) 1987

Case, Betty Jean, *Living Without Your Twin*, Tibbutt Publishing (Portland, Oregon) 1993

Case, Betty Jean, *We are Twins, But Who Am I?*, Tibbutt Publishing (Portland, Oregon) 1991

Crystal, David, *The Cambridge Encyclopaedia of Language*, Cambridge University Press (Cambridge) 1987

Douglas, Jo and Richman, Naomi, *My Child Won't Sleep*, Penguin (London) 1984

Farmer, Penelope (ed), *Two, or The Book of Twins and Doubles: an autobiographical anthology*, Little, Brown (London) 1996

Friedrich, Elizabeth and Rowland, Cherry, *The Twins Handbook: from pre-birth to first schooldays*, Robson Books (London) 1985

Green, Christopher and Chee, Kit, *Understanding Attention Deficit Disorder*, Vermilion (London) 1995

Haslam, David, *Sleepless Children*, Futura (London) 1985

Kohn, Ingrid and Moffitt, Perrin-Lynn, *Pregnancy Loss: a Silent Sorrow,* Hodder & Stoughton (London) 1995

McFadyen, Anne, *Special Care Babies and their Developing Relationships*, Routledge (London) 1995

Rosambeau, Mary, *How Twins Grow Up*, Bodley Head (London) 1987

Sandbank, Audrey, *Twins and the Family*, TAMBA and Arrow Books (London) 1988

Watson, Peter, *Twins*, Hutchinson (London) 1981

RESOURCES

Useful Addresses

TAMBA (Twins and Multiple
Birth Foundation)
P.O. Box 30
Little Sutton
South Wirral L66 1TH
Tel. 0151 348 0020

TAMBA Twinline
Tel. 01732 868000
Weekday evenings 7 pm – 11 pm
Weekends 10 am – 11 pm

MBF (Multiple Birth
Foundation)
Queen Charlotte's and Chelsea
Hospital
Goldhawk Road
London W6 0XG
Tel. 0181 748 3519

Action on Pre-Eclampsia
(APEC)
31–33 College Road
Harrow
Middx HA1 1EJ
Tel. 01923 266778
(24-hour helpline)

Association for Post-Natal Illness
25 Jerdan Place
London SW6 1BE
Tel. 0171 386 0868

Child Accident Prevention Trust
Fourth floor
Clerks Court
18–20 Farringdon Lane
London EC1R 3AU
Tel. 0171 608 3828

Child Bereavement Trust
(video and publications but
no personal support for those
outside S. Bucks)
Harleyford Estate
Henley Road
Marlow
Bucks SL7 2DX
Tel. 01628 488101

Child Death Helpline
York House
Great Ormond Street
London WC1N 3JH
Tel. 0800 282986

Compassionate Friends
(for parents whose children have
died)
53 North Street
Bristol BS3 1EN
Tel. 0117 9539639

Contact-a-Family
(information and support to
parents of special-needs children,
including those with rare
disorders)
170 Tottenham Court Road
London W1P 0HA
Tel. 0171 383 3555

CRY-SIS
(help for parents of crying
babies)
BM CRY-SIS
London WC1N 3XX
Tel. 0171 404 5011

Foundation for the Study of
Infant Deaths
14 Halkin Street
London SW1X 7DP
Tel. 0171 235 0965 (office)
Tel. 0171 235 1721 (helpline)

Harris Birthright Research
Centre (research into fetal
medicine and antenatal testing)
King's College School of
Medicine
Denmark Hill
London SE5 8RX
Tel. 0171 924 0714

Home Start UK (national
network of parents offer help to
families of young children)
2 Salisbury Road
Leicester LE1 7QR
Tel. 0116 2339955

Hyperactive Children's Support
Group
71 Whyke Lane, Chichester
West Sussex PO19 2LD
Tel. 01903 725182

La Leche League (advice and
information to women wanting
to breast-feed)
BM 3424
London WC1N 3XX
Tel. 0171 242 1278

Lone Twin Network
PO Box 5653
Birmingham B29 7JY

MAMA (Meet-A-Mum
Association; network to allevi-
ate the isolation of mothers)
Cornerstone House
14 Willis Road
Croydon CR0 2XX
Tel. 0181 665 0357

Maternity Alliance (campaigns
for better maternity benefits,
services, rights and information
to pregnant women at work)
45 Beech Street, Barbican
London EC2P 2LX
Tel. 0171 588 8583 (office)
Tel. 0171 588 8582 (helpline)

Miscarriage Association
c/o Clayton Hospital
Northgate
Wakefield
W. Yorks WF1 3JS
Tel. 01924 200799

National Childbirth Trust (NCT)
Alexandra House
Oldham Terrace
London W3 6NH
Tel. 0181 992 8637

National Council for One-Parent
Families
255 Kentish Town Road
London NW5 2LX
Tel. 0171 267 1361

Parentline (help for parents under
stress)
Endway House
The Endway
Hadleigh
Essex SS7 2AN
Tel. 01702 559900 (helpline)

Parents at Work (information on
childcare and employment rights)
45 Beech Street
Barbican
London EC2Y 8AD
Tel. 0171 628 3565

Relaxation for Living Trust
12 New Street
Chipping Norton
Oxon OX7 5LJ
Tel. 01608 646100

Royal Society for the Prevention
of Accidents (RoSPA)
Edgbaston Park
353 Bristol Road
Birmingham B5 7ST
Tel. 0121 248 2000

Support Around Termination for
Abnormality (SATFA)
73–75 Charlotte Street
London W1P 1LB
Tel. 0171 631 0280 (office)
Tel. 0171 631 0285 (helpline)

Stillbirth and Neonatal Death
Society (SANDS)
28 Portland Place
London W1N 4DE
Tel. 0171 436 7940 (office)
Tel. 0171 436 5881 (helpline)

Other Resources

Triplet and Quad Pushchairs

Gordon's Production Services
58 Cavendish Road
Salford
Greater Manchester M27 4NQ
Tel. 0161 740 9979

Petrena Products
16 The Halfcroft
Syston
Leicester LE7 8LD
Tel. 0116 2605966

INDEX

Page numbers in *italic* refer to the illustrations